A Note on the Author

Jessica Hepburn is one of the UK's leading voices on fertility, infertility and IVF. She is the author of the book *The Pursuit of Motherhood* and writes and speaks widely in the press and media on the subject of assisted conception and alternative routes to parenthood. In 2016, following her ten-year tenure as executive director of the Lyric Theatre Hammersmith, she founded Fertility Fest, the world's first arts festival dedicated to the science of making babies and modern families. In 2018 she was nominated as one of Amnesty International's Women of Suffragette Spirit and won the Fertility Foundation's inaugural Fertility Hero Award for her campaigning work.

www.jessicahepburn.com

Also by the author
The Pursuit of Motherhood

21 MILES

Swimming in Search of the Meaning of Motherhood

Jessica Hepburn

unbound

First published in 2018
This paperback edition first published in 2019

Unbound
6th Floor Mutual House, 70 Conduit Street, London W1S 2GF

www.unbound.com

Text Design by PDQ Digital Media Solutions, Bungay UK

A CIP record for this book is available from the British Library

ISBN 978-1-78352-855-4 (trade pbk)
ISBN 978-1-78352-609-3 (trade hbk)
ISBN 978-1-78352-611-6 (ebook)
ISBN 978-1-78352-610-9 (limited edition)

Printed and bound in Great Britain by Clays Ltd, Elcograf S.p.A.

'To me the sea is like a person –
like a child that I've known a long time'

Gertrude Ederle,
the first woman to swim twenty-one miles
across the English Channel

A Note from the Author

The events and interviews in this book largely took place in 2014 and 2015. It felt important to remain true to the story as it unfolded so they are recorded as they happened in the knowledge that the world changes and people's lives move on.

CONTENTS

Prologue

I slide off the side into the deep end. My body feels weightless in the water as I start to swim. Breaststroke arms and legs pull me forward; it feels like my speed is strong. Could the duckling have turned into a swan?

My opponent's mum nods admiringly as I reach the shallow end, as if she is impressed. My mum stifles a smile, I think, I can never be sure with my mum. Whoever wins today's swim-off will compete in the inter-schools swimming gala. The teachers haven't been able to decide which one of us is faster, so me and a classmate have been sent to the local pool to sprint it out, two girls marshalled by their mothers.

My opponent climbs down the steps into the water and now we are both poised, ready to start. Her mum says 'Go!' My mum stands silently watching. I'm not sure she would know what to say; she's not like most people's mums. I push off and swim, reaching ahead, pulling the water past me, kicking back. But I don't feel as quick as I did on my first length. I'm fighting the water, I'm losing the race and the coveted place in the gala.

When you're a child, life is all about speed. Who will be the first and the fastest? When you grow up, you realise that life's really about endurance. Water would teach me that.

'Can we have the works tonight?'

'You mean starter *and* pudding?'

'Go on. It is Christmas.'

'But you know I don't like puddings,' Peter says. 'I'm happy for you to have one though.'

'It's not the same eating a pudding on your own. Will you at least share one with me?'

'If it makes you feel better, I'll share one with you and *you* can eat it.'

There's no point continuing this conversation. I'm not going to win.

It's the night before Christmas Eve and we're having supper at our favourite restaurant, just round the corner from our flat. The place is fairly quiet. Most work parties are over, and everyone is either doing last-minute shopping or staying home in preparation for the excess to come. The waiter comes over.

'Shall we?' Peter asks.

'Why not? It *is* Christmas.'

'Touché,' he says, before turning to the waiter. 'Two Negronis, please.'

The waiter smiles. Every waiter who knows their

cocktails always does when you order a Negroni. It's a drink lover's drink.

I order the food. Crab on toast, followed by seven-hour lamb and a bottle of the Douro. It's what we always have.

'Any sides?' the waiter asks.

'Greens definitely,' I reply. 'Do you think we need potatoes?'

'Depends how hungry you are. The lamb's for three so it's going to be a big portion for the two of you anyway.'

'It's OK,' Peter says, 'She likes big portions.' He smiles at the waiter.

Peter likes food too. Not quite as much as me, maybe. But I could never have stayed with a man for twelve years who didn't like to eat. Having said that, my perfect partner would share my love of carbohydrates – Peter thinks they're boring.

Our Negronis arrive. 'Here's to Christmas,' he says as we clink glasses. 'And to a great year ahead.'

'You say that every year and we still haven't had one. I've been thinking about doing my own version of the Queen's Speech on Christmas Day – *2013: my annus horribilis.* I might think it was something to do with the number thirteen, except that every year for the past nine years has been unlucky.'

It was Christmas day nine years ago that Peter and I first decided to try for a baby. I had just turned thirty-four and the topic had been under discussion for a while. I'll always remember him looking at me across the dinner table, surrounded by our family, and mouthing: 'Let's do it!' But nine years later we still haven't had one. This is the first Christmas in years that we've spent at home in London. We usually escape somewhere hot, somewhere we're not reminded of the children we haven't got.

'It *is* going to be great,' Peter says in his most encouraging voice. 'This is the year you officially become a writer.'

'Yeah, but who's going to want to read a book called *The Pursuit of Motherhood* that doesn't end with a baby?'

'Not yet. There's still hope.'

'Peter, I love you for your optimism, but I've just turned forty-three. Haven't you heard that's the age a woman's fertility jumps off Beachy Head?'

'Why Beachy Head?' he says.

'Well, I would say "falls off a cliff", but apparently good writers steer clear of clichés.'

He laughs.

'Mind you,' I continue, 'clichés are clichés for a reason. They say it how it is. There's nothing active about the decline in my fertility. It's falling, not jumping.'

Peter gives me that look which I know means he's afraid I'm heading down the path of despondency. 'I don't know what you're worried about,' he says, trying to turn the conversation around, 'misery memoirs are all the rage these days.'

'Yeah, misery memoirs that have a happy ending. I know I didn't manage it by the end of the book but I was at least hoping that by the time it came out I'd be able to announce I was pregnant. It would have made a perfect real-life epilogue.'

A month earlier, just before my forty-third birthday, we had undergone another round of IVF. As usual, everything seemed to go well. Three high-quality embryos that had been fertilised 'in vitro' were put back into my womb, and we were due to find out whether I had got pregnant just before my birthday. Talk about timing: my book about our long struggle to conceive is due to come out in the new year, and it ends with me saying that I am going to continue trying for a baby until I reach the age of forty-three. This is based on the philosophy of a good friend of mine from university who'd once said to me: 'It's all about the number forty-three. If you haven't had a baby by then, you can get on with the rest of your life.' It had become my mantra, and on the eve of said birthday it felt like we had been cast in our very own version of *The Truman Show* and someone somewhere had decided to give us the most climactic happy ending. I was convinced it would be twins. I could do twins. I could even do triplets. But the cycle was negative. All we added to our family was another fifteen grand of debt and disappointment.

I pick up my glass and take another sip of Negroni.

'Let's face it,' I say, 'there's basically no chance of Julia Roberts playing me now. Who would adapt a book into a film about a woman who desperately wants a baby, does everything possible to get one, and fails?'

'Isn't she a bit old?'

'Who?'

'Julia Roberts.'

'No. Celebrities are the only people who are never too old to have babies.'

5

Our crab on toast arrives. Peter does his usual, picking off the meat and leaving the bread. It's such a waste, but with lamb for three (plus potatoes) on the way, eating his toast would be, well, greedy.

'So while we're working out what to do next, why don't you focus on all the incredible women who didn't have children?' Peter says. 'You know, like Virginia Woolf, Frida Kahlo . . .'

He's doing that optimist thing again.

'Virginia Woolf killed herself, remember,' I say.

'A minor detail. The important thing to remember is that history is full of women who didn't have children and no one thinks about whether they were mothers or not. We think about what else they did in their lives.'

'I'm not sure about that,' I reply, 'but it is true that if I can't be a mother I'm going to have to do something big instead. Something *really impressive*.'

Peter sighs. 'That's not what I meant. You don't need to try and become the next Virginia Woolf or Frida Kahlo if you don't have a baby. Why don't you just start by planning the other things you want to do in your life – like that trip you've always wanted to take on the Trans-Siberian Railway, something like that.' He pushes his plate away, toast untouched. 'God, I wish I'd never mentioned them now.'

'Trans-Mongolian,' I say pointedly.

'Pardon?'

'Trans-Mongolian Railway I want to go from Moscow to Beijing, not Vladivostok.'

'Well, Trans-whatever-it-is. What I mean is you don't need to change the world just because you can't have a baby.'

'So what's the point of being here then? If you don't have children and your only purpose is to serve the economy and maybe have a bit of fun from time to time, is it really worth it? Unless you do something Big.'

He gives me a weary look as the waiter comes over to take our plates.

'I've always fancied becoming prime minister,' I say, pouring us each a glass of wine. 'PM Hepburn, that would be pretty cool.'

'But you don't know anything about politics. You didn't even vote in the last election.'

'Yeah, well, that's because I don't know whose side I'm on any more. Maybe I could be an independent. There are definitely a few things I'd like to campaign for: three-day weekends, free public transport, the death of Starbucks . . .'

Peter laughs.

'The problem is,' I continue, 'I'm not sure anyone would vote in an "infertile" to run the country. Not when babies are what win elections.'[1]

'I hate that word. I wish you wouldn't use it.'

'What word?'

'Infertile. You're not infertile, you've been pregnant lots of times.'

'I'm not sure it counts if you don't end up with a baby.'

'Well, I'm sure you'll think of something.'

I'm thinking as our main course arrives.

'Maybe I could write another book?'

'What about?' Peter says as he starts to dish out the lamb onto our plates, well practised in putting more on mine than his own.

'About what happens next. A bit like the "Katy" series?' I say. 'You know, *What Katy Did*; *What Katy Did Next* – the books by Susan Coolidge? Didn't you read them?'

'I'm a boy. Boys don't read books about Katy.'

'Oh yeah, they prefer pictures of Katie Price.'

He gives me a look of disdain. I take two potatoes and push the bowl towards him but he ignores it.

'So, that's it,' he says. 'Write a book about *What Jessica Did Next*. Maybe she can even go to Beijing . . .' he says. 'But here's the deal: this book. I'm not in.'

'What do you mean?' I say, picking up my fork.

'I mean what I just said, I don't want to be in it.'

'You've got to be in it. Otherwise people will wonder what's happened to you. You can't just disappear.'

'Yes, I can.'

'But everyone that's read a proof of my book says you come across as a really nice guy. That's the beauty of fiction.'

'I *am* a nice guy. Your book isn't fiction. It's non-fiction. It's about our life.'

'Yeah, well you can't say that and then say that scene I wrote where we had a row is embellished.'

'Well, it was.'

'Well, maybe that's the thing about reality. It's subjective. You think that row is embellished. I don't. I chose to write you as a nice guy. It doesn't necessarily mean you are one.'

Peter looks at me. 'Either way, I still don't want to be in

it. I agreed to be in your first book because you needed to write it. But that's it. In book terms, we're getting a divorce.'

I'm quiet for a few moments.

'OK, I get you. How about a dessert instead, then? They've got Christmas pudding ice cream on the menu. If we're going to get a divorce, surely you can't deny me a scoop of ice cream?'

A List

On 1 January, I take out my New Year Resolutions Book, open a fresh page and write at the top:

1. Give up IVF and do something big instead.

I love lists. I collect them like other people collect stamps. I keep my most prized lists in small colourful notebooks stacked carefully by the side of my bed. I've got lists of all the books I've read, all the films I've seen, all the countries I've visited. And this: my New Year Resolutions Book, which I write in ceremoniously each year.

I think for a moment and then add:

2. Achieve (and stay at) my target weight of just under ten stone.

This resolution is a making a repeat appearance. For someone who loves food as much as I do it's a constant struggle. Some of the greatest moments of my life have involved me and a plate. But like many women I also long to be thin, so it goes on the list every year. And I do mean thin, not slim. Slim has always seemed to me to be on the slow slide to voluptuous – maybe it's something to do with the curvature of the letter 'S' – and everyone knows that voluptuous is only a doughnut away from being fat. Quite what I would do about this perennial resolution if I did manage to get pregnant, I'm not sure. But welcome to my confused world, where success has been all about getting fat and staying thin.

———————

Since our supper before Christmas, I have been thinking a lot about women who have done something big with their lives, and on the afternoon of New Year's Day I decide I'm going to start a new list: a list of twenty women who have changed the world. When I've done it I'm going to look up whether they had children or not. It's like my own private game. The rules are that there will be no peeking until I've finished. It beats watching football on the telly.

In order to hone the list I have had to make a few decisions. First, I've decided that to make it on you've got to be dead. I've always thought those magazine articles and TV programmes detailing the 'One hundred greatest something-or-others of all time' are misleading because they often include people or things which are just fashionable. Right now, for example, you'll find that Kate Middleton appears on a lot of lists of the most important women in history. I don't want to make assumptions, but surely it's a bit early to confer this status on her? Besides, she's alive. I told you: alive people don't count.

I've also decided to have different categories. By that I mean I'm not allowing myself too many women who've done the same sort of thing. When you start playing this game, you realise that there are so many more famous female political leaders and writers than there are, for example, composers and scientists. Arguably, those people who have made a mark in fields where women are under-represented have done something even more significant. Not that this list is about value judgements, but you've got to have criteria, otherwise how do you begin?

Oh, and there's just one more thing before I do the big reveal: I'm allowing myself to include both Virginia Woolf and Frida Kahlo, even though I already know that neither of them had children. They would probably have made the list anyway – especially Frida Kahlo, as visual art is another area where there is a dearth of famous historical female figures. But as this is my list and I'm in charge, I've made the decision to give myself a golden hello. After all, I don't want to find out that my list of top twenty women changed history *and* they were all mothers – that's just not going to help my state of mind right now. I need at least a few women who I know I can rely on.

By teatime the list is complete:

Writers
1. Sappho
2. Jane Austen
3. Virginia Woolf

Artists/Designers

4. Frida Kahlo
5. Coco Chanel

Composers/Musicians

6. Ella Fitzgerald
7. Édith Piaf

Actresses

8. Hepburn, Audrey and Katharine
9. Marilyn Monroe

World Leaders

10. Cleopatra
11. Boudicca
12. Joan of Arc
13. Queen Elizabeth I and Queen Victoria
14. Margaret Thatcher

Political and Social Activists

15. Mary Wollstonecraft
16. Emmeline Pankhurst

Humanitarian Figures

17. Florence Nightingale
18. Mother Teresa

Scientists

19. Marie Curie

Cooks/Chefs
20.   Isabella (Mrs) Beeton (well, the world's got to eat!)

OK, I realise that there are a couple of cheats here: I've included two names at number eight, but as Katharine and Audrey regularly top best-ever actress lists and both share my surname, I'm going to take author's ancestral licence and include them as a single entry (not that we're directly related, but there must be some kind of link). And, yes, number thirteen, too, but if you're going for a British royal, how do you choose between these two?

With the list complete, I start to research who had children. The good news is that my two cheats actually cancel each other out, so I don't need to feel bad about those. Katharine Hepburn didn't have children but Audrey did. Likewise, Elizabeth, the virgin queen, had none, and Victoria had nine. Sadly, I think I'm going to have to omit the ancient Greek writer Sappho – not from the list, per se, but from the statistics. Some sources say she had a daughter but so little is known about her life that's it impossible to be sure. The fact that she is one of the first known 'lesbians' – she came from the island of Lesbos, the origin of the term – is irrelevant. It certainly doesn't preclude the ability, desire or right to become a mother.

Also cancelling each other out, or at the very least making things complicated, are my two musicians. Ella Fitzgerald never had children herself but adopted her half-sister's son, whom she named Ray Brown Jr after her husband and then gave to another of her sisters to bring up. And Édith Piaf did have a daughter, Marcelle, who was taken away from her as a baby and died of meningitis at just two years old.

So where does that leave me? Well, on the writer front, Jane Austen, like Virginia Woolf, never had children. And Coco Chanel, like Frida Kahlo, didn't either. Nor did Marilyn Monroe. In terms of world leaders, Cleopatra did. In fact, sources say she had four, which bemuses me because I always think of her doomed love affair with Antony, which had no hope of any progeny. Boudicca (or Boadicea, as I was taught to call her) apparently had children too, despite her warring preoccupations. As did Margaret Thatcher (who had twins). But Joan of Arc, who was about nineteen when she died on that stake, was way too busy saving France and making sure she became a saint to think about motherhood. Mary Wollstonecraft and Emmeline Pankhurst, two of the leading figures in the women's movement, both had children; in fact Mary died as a result of complications during the labour of her second child. But notably Florence Nightingale and Mother Teresa, who were arguably much more maternal figures, did not (although admittedly Mother Teresa was a nun). Marie Curie was a mother. So was Mrs Beeton. Of course she was. What else would you expect from such an archetypal homemaker – a mother of eight, she adopted her husband's four children from his first marriage and then had four more of her own.

So the results are in. After I've eliminated the don't-knows, the cancelled-outs and any other complications, I discover that over half of the women on my list didn't have children. Given that the vast majority of women in the world do – and the percentage was even higher in the past – it's a staggering statistic. In fact, on the basis of my list, you could go so far as to say that if you're a woman and you're going to do something big, you're more likely than not to be childless.

For a moment I feel excited that I'm in such good company. But then I feel something else: a pain all too familiar. Because what I really want to know is whether it was enough for these women that they did something with their lives which has resonated for generations to come. Or did they, deep down, wish they had been mothers?

Blue Monday

Monday morning, mid-January. The weather is cold, grey, resolutely Januaryish. I get on the tube to work and open the paper to see an article that says it's officially the most depressing day of the year. Blue Monday, it's called. I look at the people sitting around me. The obligatory person listening to music too loudly on their headphones. A woman playing a game on her phone in which she seems to be doing something, I don't know what, with colourful shapes. Another woman with electric-blue eyeliner staring into space. And a man sitting opposite me who is reading *The Unbearable Lightness of Being*. The cover looks new; perhaps he was given it for Christmas.

I wonder how they're all feeling inside. Are they depressed? Are they dreaming of doing something big with their lives too?

The tube pulls slowly into Hammersmith. I've been coming to the same station for over a decade, longer even than I've been trying to have a baby. I run a theatre here. Not an operating theatre – one with a stage where people perform. This distinction has become important over the last few years, given the amount of time I've spent with fertility doctors, lying on trolleys with my feet in the air. Whenever they ask me what I do, their eyes light up in recognition, until I correct them.

I know that the people I work with will be surprised and shocked at the lengths I've gone to to try and conceive. Publicly, I am a successful 'career woman' (that terrible term which is never used to describe men) but privately I've been desperately trying to become a mother. For years I've done my utmost to avoid detection, arranging clinic appointments wherever possible before and after work. Even when going through IVF treatment, I'd have my eggs collected under general anaesthetic in the morning and be back at my desk by lunch. I know I can't be the only woman to have done this. They say that around one in six couples struggle to conceive. I don't know how they get these statistics but if it's true it's happening on every street in every town. Yet most people don't talk about it, not openly or often anyway, because infertility is a stigma still shrouded in secrecy and shame. And now I've gone and written about it and everyone is going to know the full horror.

I walk out of the station, cross the road with the crowds and head into Pret to pick up some breakfast. I hover by the fruit salad for a moment and then think, bugger it, and get a croissant and a coffee.

My first meeting of the day is a long and tedious one. We're building an extension to the theatre and the costs are getting too high. We are going through each item, line by line, to try and bring the budget down. I'm surrounded by men in suits who work on the management side of the construction industry and are getting frustrated with me because I refuse to compromise on how nice I want the new toilets to be. Unfortunately for them, I raised the money for this project and am paying their extortionate fees, so they can't ignore me. As they tap on their calculators, comparing the cost of full-height versus half-height tiling, my mind wanders,

I can't help thinking that feminism has a lot to answer for. Of course I wouldn't say that if Mary Wollstonecraft or Emmeline Pankhurst were in the room. But they're not, they're dead, so I figure I'm all right. Nor do I want to seem ungrateful for everything they did to help liberate women from being seen only as wives and mothers. It's because of them that I am educated and have the right to vote (even if I've not always been very good at using it). In fact, you could say it's because of them that I am sitting here now and these men are ultimately going to have to listen to my views on tiling, because I already know I'm not going to compromise. But even though Mary and Emmeline unquestionably achieved something big for me and all of womankind, I do feel there is something that they never fully grappled with, and that is this: *nature is not a feminist.*

Like many women of my generation, I didn't ever consider that I would have a baby before my thirties. I went to an all-girls comprehensive school in north London renowned for turning out independent, go-getting young women. We were all encouraged to attend university and get on the career ladder in our twenties. The limited sex education we received was mainly focused on how not to have a baby. Teenage pregnancy equalled disaster, or so we were led to believe. No one was supposed to settle down with the first boy they kissed, it was good to be picky, and every girl was looking for the perfect modern man. In fact, motherhood wasn't much discussed at all. It was certainly never presented as a career path, and for those of us who knew we wanted to have children, we just assumed it would happen as and when we were ready.

This would be fine if everything went to plan. But if you're a woman and you get to your thirties before deciding to have a baby, and you then find that getting pregnant isn't as easy as you thought it would be – as you were told it would be – time is suddenly running out. Because the thing we're not told at school, or at least not explicitly, is that a woman is born with her lifetime supply of eggs, and day by day, from puberty, these eggs diminish in number and quality as she gets older. This essentially means that the longer you wait, the harder it's going to be to conceive. It doesn't mean you can't and won't get pregnant – in fact because so many people are leaving it later, the average age of first-time mothers is increasing, and there are definitely social and economic benefits to becoming a parent later in life. But any good doctor will tell you that the optimum biological age for a woman to have children is around twenty-five; if you leave it until your thirties or forties, it might not happen as easily, and there will be less time to sort out any problems if you have them. Because even though life expectancy is increasing – another reason that later parenthood is not necessarily a bad thing – the average age of the female menopause has not changed, and around ten years before a woman reaches it, her chance of giving birth to her own biological baby massively diminishes. That age is generally around forty-three, but the hard truth is your fertility has actually been falling off Beachy Head since puberty; that's just the age when it hits the sea.

Forty-three is a prime number. It has its own Wikipedia page. It is also a centred heptagonal, a Heegner and a repdigit. Forty-three is the atomic number for technetium, a silvery grey metal. It is the international dialling code for Austria, the name of a Spanish liqueur and the number of the bus route that goes from Barnet to London Bridge. Now I am forty-three, and like all prime numbers I seem to be divisible by only one, and that one is me. Like I said, nature is not a feminist. And maybe that's why the number of women entering their forties childless has doubled in a generation. If these women are anything like me, it's not necessarily because they've actively chosen not to have children – many of them probably assumed they would be mothers too, and now they're left wondering what the hell they're going to do.

———

It's hard to explain the pain of losing something you never had. Something that was never more than an expectation, a dream or at most a cluster of cells. It's not like I'm dying or we're on the verge of a humanitarian disaster. People don't need to start having sex to save the human race because I can't have children. I know it's a hole in my life that society finds difficult to understand. I call it the pain of never, and these are its symptoms. If you've got them, you'll know.

Never feeling like a real woman because you can't do what every other woman seemingly finds so easy to do;

Never being able to feel happy for someone when they announce they're pregnant without feeling sad for yourself at the same time;

Never being able to admit that you've been in the loo crying about it because you don't want people to pity you;

Never being invited to a baby shower, christening or children's party without it hurting;

Never not being invited to a baby shower, christening or children's party because people are trying to spare your feelings without that hurting even more;

Never being able to make a pregnancy announcement to your family and friends and have them throw their arms around you in warm congratulations;

Never being able to legitimately eat for two or buy a cool maternity dress or go into a bookstore and buy *What to Expect When You're Expecting* (although I did once and then I miscarried and felt like a fraud);

Never feeling the first kick of life inside you;

Never being able to say, 'I think my waters have
     broken', or 'Bring me gas and air.' Is that what
     people really say? Never knowing that;
Never having a baby placed on your chest and
     saying 'hello' for the first time;
Never being able to breastfeed and use your
     body for what it was built for;
Never being able to write an 'out of office' that
     says 'I'm away on maternity leave';
Never being able to see your child's first steps;
Or first words;
Or first day at school;
Or first anything;
Never being able to share these things with your
     friends, and growing distant because of it;
Never seeing someone else's photos of their
     children on Facebook without wishing you
     had photos to post too;
Never hearing anyone call you 'Mum'

That's the pain of never.

———

Later in the day, when I'm back at my desk eating lunch,
checking my emails and feeling good that I won the War
of the Tiles, I overhear some colleagues chatting. Someone
they know parachuted out of a plane over the weekend
to raise money for Cancer Research. Everyone starts

comparing personal fundraising challenges. Someone says they want to run the London Marathon next year; someone else wants to walk the Coast to Coast.

'Hey, Jessica,' they shout across the room. 'What would you do for charity?'

'I don't know,' I say. 'I've never done a sponsored anything.'

'You should do a sponsored swim,' someone says.

Everyone laughs.

'Pardon?' I say, my mouth full of ham and cheese.

'A few lengths up and down the pool, surely you could manage that?'

Everyone laughs again.

'What's so funny?' I say. It's true I've never been known for my athletic prowess and I don't look good in a swimming costume, but who does?

For the rest of the afternoon I can't get the conversation out of my head. It's reminded me that several years ago, when Peter and I were away on holiday after another IVF failure, I'd started a new list book: my Bucket List Book. Top of the first page was 'Become a mother'. But there were other things on the list as well. Positioned between 'Get a cat' and 'Learn to stand on my head', I'd written something down that had been a long-forgotten childhood dream. I hadn't thought about it for nearly thirty years when I wrote it and, if I'm honest, I hadn't thought about it again since. If number one on my bucket list had come to fruition, then it would probably have been consigned to list history.

Yet in that moment, on Blue Monday afternoon, as

everyone laughs, it suddenly comes back to me. It's big. It's not the sort of thing you could do with a toddler in tow.

That will teach them, I think.

I pick up the phone to call Peter. And then I remember. I'm not allowed to here. He doesn't want to be in this story.

Horizontal Walking

'Hi, is that John?' I say into the receiver.

'Yes.'

'I found your details on the internet. I was wondering whether you might be able to help me?'

'I'll try,' he says gamely. His voice is positively plummy.

I take a moment before speaking.

'I think I want to swim the English Channel . . .'

'Do you?' he says. 'What makes you think that?'

'It's a childhood dream,' I say and then add: 'Turned mid-life crisis.'

He breaks into a chuckle. 'If you don't mind me asking, how old are you?' he says.

'Forty-three.'

'And are you a swimmer?'

'Well, I can swim. I wouldn't call myself *a* swimmer.'

'Did you swim competitively as a child? For your county or a club?'

'No.'

'Have you ever done any open-water swimming before?'

'No.'

'Well, how many times a week do you swim?'

I pause, wondering whether this is the sort of moment that justifies a fib. I don't want him to write me off already, but since I started trying to get pregnant I've all but given up exercise. There's a theory that doing too much isn't helpful when trying to conceive and, whilst I don't think this means you're supposed to abandon it altogether, up against all the other things you're told to give up – alcohol, coffee, etc. – this wasn't a hard one for me. In fact, it was really rather easy. I've never been very good at sport, and the only thing I really like about exercising is feeling virtuous when it's over. At school, I was the sort of person who had to suffer the ignominy of being last to be picked for the rounders team. But I did enjoy swimming when I was a child, and not just because we always went to McDonald's on the way home. For years I attended a swimming class on a Wednesday night at the Prince of Wales Road baths in Kentish Town. The instructor, Max, in his black trunks and red terry-towelling T-shirt, would line us all up along the pool in speed order. I was always towards the back. Everyone used to joke that my best stroke was breaststroke legs.

Then one day, when I didn't get into the school swimming team (again), I found myself consoling my dad. It was always harder managing his disappointment than my own, so I told him that it didn't matter that I hadn't got in, because one day I was going to swim the Channel instead. I think I must have read about someone doing it in a newspaper, and I figured you didn't need to be fast to swim all the way to France – you just needed to be able to keep going. I've always been good at keeping going. That's probably why I've done eleven rounds of IVF. (Yes, that's right, eleven. I didn't want to mention the number before because I thought it might appal you.)

I refocus my thoughts on the question at the other end of the phone line. 'Maybe once a week,' I say and then add, 'on average.'

This is a semi-fib. I can up my average if I include holidays, but it's probably more like once a month (if that). Sometimes I don't even swim between holidays.

'Can you crawl?'

For a moment I'm confused by the baby reference before I realise what he's asking.

'I can do the crawl. Well, a few lengths. I'm much better at breaststroke.'

'The problem with breaststroke is you'll have to be in the water longer. One of the main challenges of the Channel is the cold. The aim is to get over to the other side and out as quickly as possible.'

'Doesn't a wetsuit help with the cold?'

'I'm afraid you can't wear one of those. Not if you want to be an official Channel swimmer.'

This is news to me, and it isn't good. I hate the cold, possibly even more than I hate exercise. In fact, one of my main mottos in life is: 'You can never be too cosy.'

John goes on to explain that wetsuits hadn't been invented in 1875 when the Englishman Captain Matthew Webb became the first person to swim the Channel. The rules state that you have to remain true to that tradition today, and can only don a costume, hat and goggles.

'Right,' I respond slowly, taking in all the information he's given me. 'So how far is it and how long does it take?'

'Twenty-one miles. It takes around fifteen hours on average. But you'll be adding another five to ten hours if you want to do it breaststroke.'

There's a beat of silence.

'Fifteen hours?' I say, trying not to sound too incredulous.

'That's right. It's a long way to France.'

I pause as I take in the enormity of what he's just said.

'Well, I guess at least I can stay in a nice hotel when I get there and have croissants in bed for breakfast.'

He chuckles again. Actually, it's more like a guffaw.

'You can't stay in France,' he says.

'Why?'

'You don't go through passport control when you're swimming the Channel. As soon as you touch land, you pick up a pebble and then you're back on the boat to England.'

'You mean I won't even get a croissant?'

'No,' he laughs. 'But I wouldn't worry about that. If you do swim the Channel, you won't want to move or eat anything for at least a week.'

'No?'

'No.'

'That bad, huh?'

'That bad.'

I don't quite know what to say next. I'm starting to think this wasn't the right big idea after all. I half-heartedly enquire about the training camps John organises for aspiring Channel swimmers, which were the reason for my call. He tells me that he's running one in Formentera, a little island off Ibiza, in a couple of months for people who are doing their six-hour qualifier. I tentatively ask what this means, dreading the answer, and he tells me you need to be certified as having swum six hours in water below sixteen degrees Celsius before you can attempt the Channel.

'You mean you can't just go down to the south coast on a nice day and start splashing?'

He laughs. 'Why don't you come along and see how you get on?'

'OK, I'll have a think about it,' I say. 'It sounds good.'

I'm just saying that. It doesn't sound good. It sounds hard. I put down the phone feeling slightly sick but then do what I can to rally myself. I've been on a six-hour walk. Surely swimming for six hours is just the same thing, but horizontal. How hard can it be?

Addicted to IVF

One of the things that is not on my bucket list is seeing my legs in a tabloid newspaper. But I woke up this morning and there they were.

I'd agreed to do the article as publicity for my book. They'd been very specific that I had to wear a dress to the photoshoot. No dark colours. No patterns. Three different people had rung over the course of twenty-four hours to remind me. I'd picked out a red dress I'd bought in an M&S sale a few years ago, one of those great buys that cost twenty quid but in a good light (I like to think) looks like it could be Chanel. When I got to the location of the shoot the photographer looked me up and down.

'Nice,' he said. 'But I'm afraid you're going to have to take those off.'

He pointed at my black tights.

'What?' I said, horrified.

'The paper only does bare legs.'

'You're joking?'

'Didn't they tell you?'

'No. They told me to wear a dress. Three times. They

didn't mention anything about tights. Once.'

'Sorry,' he said. 'No can do, I'm afraid.'

'But you don't understand, my legs never come out,' I said. 'They haven't seen sunlight in over a decade.'

'It will be fine,' he said, trying to placate me. 'We'll airbrush them if they look a bit blotchy.'

To say I was mortified would be an understatement. The whole dress business was sexist enough. The only time something similar had happened to me was when I was doing a temping job in a city law firm during my university summer holidays. At the end of the first day my boss had come up to me and said that I could come back tomorrow as long as I didn't mind wearing a skirt. If she'd been a man I might have thought it was sexual harassment, but it was just company policy. Even twenty-five years ago it seemed archaic. But this is the new millennium – is there really a national newspaper that will only photograph women in dresses (no black tights)?

I suppose, in a way, I should be pleased. After all, a dress says 'woman' in the same way that infertility says 'failed woman'. In tabloid terms the most 'womanly' woman is always a mother. They must still think there's hope. Otherwise, surely, they would have put me in a black trouser suit. On the double-page spread to the left of my head are the words: 'Addicted to IVF'. I suppose going through multiple rounds of treatment and having nothing to show for it but a cleaned-out bank account does seem like a pretty extreme habit. I look at the picture, all legs and smoky eyes, and can't quite believe it's me. For years I'd kept my struggle to have a baby a secret and now, suddenly, I've become the poster girl for infertility. It's not even as if it's going to be tomorrow's chip paper. The article is on the internet, indelible forever.

A few days ago I made a pact with myself that when the article came out I wouldn't look at the online comments. Nobody should go into that lion's den. But of course I immediately do. I scroll down and the first comment reads: 'I want a baby, kinda sums her up.' I kinda have to agree. I do want a baby. One that I have made with the man that I love and who, with any luck, will inherit the best bits of both of us. I want to introduce them to the world: read them *The Very Hungry Caterpillar* and *The Tiger Who Came to Tea*. I want to organise birthday parties with pass the parcel and musical bumps. I want to open stockings at Christmas and plan egg hunts at Easter. I want a reason to go to the zoo and make fairy cakes for tea. And on the subject of food, I want to encourage my children to love shellfish and sprouts from a very young age.

Throughout the day I watch in fascinated horror as more and more comments appear and people anonymously press the arrows beside them to indicate whether they agree or disagree. For the first time in my life I have a tiny taste of what it must be like to be a celebrity, shaped by the opinions of people who have never even met you. But overall I come out of the den fairly unscathed; sympathy for my story seems to be strong. The lions are licking my wounds, not eating me.

TV and radio interviews follow. A girl could get used to being picked up in a chauffeur-driven car. But, all things being equal, I'd much rather be singing 'The Wheels on the Bus'.

It's an extraordinary and surreal few weeks. But the most overwhelming thing of all is the messages of advice and support I start to receive from all over the world, from total strangers. They tell me about miracle doctors and recommend clinics in Spain, Greece, India and the Caribbean. They suggest I try alternative treatments I've never heard of, such as Qigong, tapping and the Peruvian maca root. In one email someone writes to me about a powerful man of God from Uganda called Brother Ronnie Makabai, who prays for infertile couples and women who are past childbearing age and then they miraculously give birth (the email adds in parenthesis, 'providing their husbands are still alive'). They share heart-lifting stories involving egg donation and adoption. And about women who have got pregnant in their mid-forties with their own eggs – one woman tells me she is forty-five and has three children under the age of five, all of whom were conceived naturally, and none of them twins. Several people even offer to be a surrogate for me. Above all everyone urges me not to give up hope – that some way, somehow, I can and must become a mother.

The concern and encouragement from so many people who have never even met me but have taken the time and trouble to write is humbling. But at the same time, as more and more messages pour in, I feel myself becoming increasingly anxious. I'd thought I'd already done everything I could to become a mother. I've been to nearly a dozen clinics and had every test known to woman and doctor in a bid to work out what's wrong. Besides multiple rounds of IVF, I've tried numerous complementary therapies including acupuncture and Chinese herbs. I've even been on an intense therapeutic process to release my 'inner child' in the hope that it would help me to conceive. Yet now I'm wondering if I've tried hard enough. Maybe I haven't tried everything. The world still believes I can be a mother, even if I'm not sure I can myself. And nobody, not a single person, writes to me and says: 'You're *forty-three*, go and do something big and have a fulfilling life without children instead.'

———

One evening, in the aftermath of the article, I'm in the kitchen making myself a cup of tea. As I wait for the kettle to do its thing I think back over the last few bewildering weeks. I feel like I'm a rope in a tug of war: pulling me from one end is motherhood, the thing I've always wanted but had almost given up believing I could have, and on the other end an alternative future doing something big and finding meaning in motherlessness. I feel taut with fear at giving either one of them the advantage.

I open the cupboard to get out a teabag and spot a large bar of Green & Black's white chocolate that I bought the other day when I was feeling chocolatey, but had then foregone when I got home for a large packet of salt and vinegar Kettle Chips instead. I know the chocolate is unlikely to stand any chance of survival if I open it, but I did weigh myself yesterday and I'd lost two pounds last week so I decide to take the risk. I head into the sitting room with my cup of tea and the chocolate, sit down on the sofa and open my laptop. A new message pops into my inbox:

> *Hello Jessica*
> *My wife read your article and wanted to know whether she could ask you where you got the red dress that you were wearing. She said it looked really amazing and wondered if she could be cheeky and ask. She doesn't have an email account so she asked if I'd mail you.*
> *Hope all goes well for you.*
> *Richard*

See what I mean – all sorts of nice messages – and at least it's not another avenue that I need to explore. I don't need any more avenues; I need a road closure. I stare at the screen, vaguely wondering what sort of woman would not have an email account and ask her husband to write to a stranger about their dress. Still, I don't want to be rude, so I take a sip of tea and a square of chocolate and hit reply. It's only then that I notice that my correspondent calls himself Robinson Crusoe and his email address is prefixed 'desertislanddick'. Thankfully, he didn't mention my legs.

Can Rolls, Can't Hepburn

As I step off the plane, I feel that rush of heat that denotes holidays and happiness. But this is different. I'm on my own. I have no idea where I'm going. I've got goggles.

I take out my mobile phone and turn off airplane mode and Movistar tinkles 'hello'. Apparently a couple of other people who are coming on the swimming tour are on the same flight as me. We've arranged to text when we arrive so we can travel together. There is no international airport on Formentera so we've had to fly to Ibiza, from where we're getting a ferry.

Texts exchanged, we convene by the airport taxi rank. There are three people in addition to me. A tall couple, Mark and Teresa, and a shorter stocky guy called Andy. They are all younger than me. But they're polite: they don't ask my age, nor whether I'm married and have children, which is such a relief because I hate that middle-age-conversation-stopper question. They do, however, ask me why I've come.

'What do you want to do that for?' Andy scoffs.

'Don't you? I thought that was why we were all here.'

'Hell no,' he says. 'I've come to lie on the beach. Do as little swimming as possible.'

'Oh,' I reply, taking in this news as I turn to the couple.

Teresa shakes her head: 'Me neither, it's much too hard, but Mark is planning to do a solo at some point. Maybe this summer if his shoulder's up to it.'

Mark explains he had an operation on it a few months ago and will be taking things easy this week too. I'm not sure whether these revelations are good news for me or not. After all, I came here on business. Channel business. These people seem to think it's a holiday.

———

As we pull into the harbour on Formentera, I can see a man standing on the jetty. This, I deduce, must be John. He looks the way he speaks: English, jovial, outdoorsy.

'Hello, chaps,' he booms. 'You made it! Good job!'

He smiles broadly and claps each of us on the back. He seems to know the others well. They call him not by his first name but by his initials, JCR, the J standing for John and the CR for his surname, Coningham-Rolls. It feels a bit familiar referring to him as an acronym so I decide that I will carry on calling him John.

John throws our things in the boot of his four-by-four and we set off. We're staying in a house on the edge of the beach a little way up the coast. It sits at the end of an unmarked gravel track, one of three whitewashed stone properties that were built in the 1950s by three different English couples.

The middle one belonged to John's grandparents and is called Can Rolls, which translates from the Spanish into 'House of the Rolls'. It makes me think of him coming from a family of the finest double-barrelled bakers.

The house has hardly been touched since it was built; it has no electricity and the water is heated by solar power. The open terrace at the front drops down into the sand and overlooks the most breathtakingly beautiful bay. I later learn that the spot is in fact so idyllic that the Spanish government has decided to consecrate it as a natural heritage site and has stipulated that all three houses will need to be pulled down in thirty years' time in order to reclaim the area for nature. The properties are so eco-friendly and sympathetic to the landscape, I can't help feeling that the government might be better placed directing its bulldozers towards the high-rises of Magaluf.

It's already past seven in the evening when we arrive. Drinks and canapés on the terrace pre-supper are mooted. But my three travelling companions decide to take a dip in the sea first. They ask me if I'd like to come too but I politely decline, saying that I'm going to unpack. I don't say what I'm really thinking, which is: 'Why don't we just get on with the drinks and canapés?'

From the window of my room, which looks out over the bay, I observe them as they stroll down to the sea, dive in and swim out to a rock that is jutting out of the water a little way away from the shore. Once there, they climb onto it and sit chatting in the setting sun. I watch in a kind of awe, realising that these people are not of my species. They are clearly at home in the sea, their strokes strong and lithe. They are the sort of people who don't question taking a dip before supper. They don't think about the salt on their skin or the fact that they'll mess up their hair. They may profess not to want to swim the Channel, or even swim very much while they're here, but they could if they wanted to. All of them. They are the sort of people who got picked for the school swimming team and have trophies on the mantelpiece and certificates on the wall.

———————

The following day, after breakfast, the whole group convenes for a briefing. John gives us an overview of the week, which basically seems to consist of upping our time and distance each day. He also gives us a safety briefing. Hypothermia and jellyfish are both mentioned. He then suggests we go round in turn and say what our ambitions for the week are. Since arriving and seeing all the other people here I have felt myself growing increasingly anxious about the whole thing. I am starting to realise that open-water swimming is a whole different ball game to doing a few laps in the pool. Not that there's a ball involved, but you know what I mean – breaststroke legs just aren't going to cut it. These people know what they're doing. I don't. So when it's my turn, the only answer I feel I can give is that I hope I'm not going to hold everyone back.

Afterwards John takes me to one side and asks if I'm OK and I confess my nervousness. 'Could I just do breaststroke?'

I ask. 'I'm not sure I'm ready to tackle too much crawl along with everything else you seem to have to deal with out there.'

'Of course,' he replies, 'take it slowly.' And then in his best booming voice, he shouts: 'Right chaps, ready to go in fifteen minutes! Get changed and don't forget to put suncream on and get vased up.'

'Vased up?' I mouth to Teresa, baffled.

'Vaseline,' she says. 'Under your straps so your costume doesn't rub.'

I nod, a whole new world opening up to me, and then head upstairs to get changed.

One by one everyone congregates on the terrace. Costumes, hats and goggles on. Suncream and Vaseline applied. Someone kindly gives me some earplugs and says it helps with the cold. I take them gratefully. We file down to the water's edge. It's a beautiful day and the sea is blue and sparkling but the beach is deserted and we have it to ourselves.

John calls us into a group: 'Right chaps, as this is our first swim, we're just going to take it easy. Twenty minutes maximum. Jessica, you start by swimming over to the rock and back. Let's take a look at your breaststroke.'

I tell myself I'll be fine. Twenty minutes of breaststroke, surely that's doable. We all start to wade into the water. The first touch on my toes is cold yet almost inviting. But as I walk further in, the sharpness of the water strikes full force and I know that this is the moment when you have to commit or lose your nerve. I fall forwards into the waves and a rush of ice surrounds me. The sky may be blue but there's a reason no one is on this beautiful beach: it's the beginning of April and the water's fucking freezing. (Apologies for the 'f' word. I did think of using the word 'flipping', it would still have made for nice alliteration, but I'm afraid it just doesn't cover it.) I start to swim, breaststroke arms and legs but with my head above the water while I acclimatise. After a few strokes I force myself to duck under and the cold envelops me further.

'Good job, Hepburn', I hear John shout. 'Over to the rock and back'.

I'm not aware of the others; they have disappeared from view. All I am conscious of is me and the cold. I plough on, knowing that the only way to get used to it is to keep swimming. The rock is only a little way off but it seems to take me ages to reach it; as I get closer the water shallows around the coral and it's difficult to avoid scraping my knees. I turn round and head back to the shore, where John is standing at the water's edge.

'Well done', he says. 'That's a nice breaststroke you've got there. Now let's have a look at your crawl'.

'What?' I splutter. This isn't what we agreed.

'How are you finding the cold?' John asks.

'Agony'.

'Well, you better get to France quickly then. Crawl's the only way to do that'.

'OK, I'll give it a go. How much longer have we got?'

'You've done ten minutes. Just swim to the end of the beach and back and then you can get out'.

'Ten minutes? Is that all?'

'Off you go. Keep swimming, otherwise you'll get cold. This is Can Rolls, remember, not Can't Hepburn'.

I set off with only one thought in my mind. I don't think I can manage fifteen minutes in water this cold, let alone fifteen hours. This Channel thing is big. It's bigger than I ever imagined.

Her Darling Child

It was a Wednesday evening when the email popped into my inbox. At 18:04, to be precise. It read:

Dear Jessica,

We will never know what Jane Austen thought about not marrying and not having a family of her own, because we have no evidence that she ever told anybody. She was certainly acutely aware of the pitfalls of an 'unequal' marriage and portrayed them in her novels, as well as the happier ones.

However, since she had endless nieces and nephews, some of whom stayed with her, some of them recorded how they loved her, and she recorded how she played with some of them, I am sure being an aunt was the next best thing to being a mother (especially when you can give them back to their parents!). She was, nevertheless, never blinded to their true natures.

She did have an offer of marriage but, despite the man having an estate and good fortune and being the brother of her friends, she turned it down because she realised that she didn't love the man. She told her favourite niece that, whilst it was good to respect a man, one should not marry without love (or the possibility of respect turning into love). She also said that it was a good thing not to marry too soon because the woman would not then be subject to so many pregnancies. She was always concerned about one of her nieces, in that respect, calling her 'a poor animal'.

It was certainly not through the lack of society, like the Brontës, that she never married – the number of people she knew, met, and wrote about is staggering; perhaps she was too picky (like some of us today!) or some men might have found her too shrewd! Who knows?

It is true that, had Jane Austen married, she would not have had the time and energy, or perhaps the inclination, to write and we would not have had all those wonderful novels. In fact she called Pride and Prejudice *'her darling child'. Whether or not the novels were sublimation, we will never know.*

Regards,

Maureen Stiller,

Hon. Secretary, Jane Austen Society

AGONY!

I've had a few catchphrases in my time, 'Is eleven too early for lunch?' being one of my particular favourites. But over the course of nearly a week in Formentera I develop a new catchphrase. Whenever I get out of the sea and am asked how I'd found it, my response is always the same: 'It was AGONY!'

Each day the time and distance in the water would rise in small increments, but there was nothing about it that was getting any easier. It only takes a few days before I resort to begging. During our afternoon swim I stand up in the shallows and shout to John that I can't go on.

'Yes you can,' he bellows back. 'Off you go, Hepburn.'

I fall forwards into the water and try to lift one arm over the other but my body is screaming. I let my feet touch the sand again.

'I can't,' I say, my voice sounding pathetically weak and whiny.

'Get back in the water,' John shouts from the shore.

'I don't think I can do it,' I moan.

'Get back in the water,' he shouts again. 'Another ten minutes and then you can get out.'

From somewhere inside me, I find the strength to swim. I start out towards the rock but after a few minutes turn back and start pacing the shoreline, constantly looking up and saying, 'Is it time yet?'

'Not yet,' John replies, and then the same thing over and over again. 'Not yet . . . Not yet . . . Not yet.' And finally: 'In you come. Good job, Hepburn. Good job.'

John's two swimming assistants, Alice and Catherine, hold out my towel as I stagger out of the water, their congratulations warm and genuine.

'It's just so hard,' I say, taking the towel gratefully and wrapping it round me.

They laugh. 'Don't you mean it was AGONY?'

———

On the penultimate morning of the tour, when I come down from my room to breakfast, John, Andy and Mark are sitting at the table eating and chatting.

'Just the person we've been talking about,' John says. 'How are you feeling today?'

'Ready for more agony,' I say cheerily.

'We've just been discussing whether you should try and do a Channel relay this summer if there's a cancellation.'

'A relay? What's that?'

'You swim the Channel as a team. Each person is in the water for one hour in succession until you get to France,' Mark explains.

'How many people in the team?'

'Usually six, but you can do it with less. Obviously, the smaller the number the more times you'll swim and the bigger test it will be. It will be a good way of seeing whether you really want to attempt a solo. What do you think?'

'I think: is my crawl up to it?'

'Well, you should have some lessons to improve your technique, but basically you just need to learn to keep going,' John says.

'And if you do a relay you'd rather be in the water than on the boat,' Andy adds.

'Why's that?' I ask.

'You get terrible seasickness on the boat.'

'Sounds like fun.'

'I told you,' Andy says. 'Swimming the Channel isn't.'

'Yup, I'm starting to realise that,' I concede.

In fact, I'm starting to learn a lot of things which are making me wonder why anyone would want to take on the challenge of the Channel. It may be twenty-one miles from Dover to Cap Gris-Nez, which is the nearest point of land in France from England, but the tides are so strong you can't swim in a straight line. Instead you zigzag across, and the distance you have to cover is much greater than that. In the past you could swim from France to England, which was considered tidally easier than the other way around, but nowadays the French have banned it. (Too much hassle or something. No doubt Joan of Arc would have been proud of them for taking a stand against the Brits.) I've also learned that there is only a small window each year when the water's warm enough to get across, and even then it's going to be cold, far below the temperature of any swimming pool. And because of all these things – the tides, the distance, the cold and the unpredictability of the weather – I've learned that a very high percentage of those who set out don't make it across. It's one of the toughest physical and mental endurance feats on the planet. Fewer people have swum the Channel than have climbed Mount Everest.

But I have also learned something else, an unexpected boon that does make it worth giving it a second thought: aspiring Channel swimmers get to eat. A lot. Apparently most people put on a couple of extra stone in the lead-up to their swim as it is by the far the best way of keeping out the cold for the longest possible time. The appropriate cliché to use here is: 'Every cloud has a silver lining', or perhaps I should say instead, 'Every wave has a chocolate coating'.

I help myself to a large bowl of cereal.

'So, John,' I say. 'What have you got in store for us today?'

'Wait and see, Hepburn,' he says cryptically. 'Wait and see.'

Try as I might, it's impossible to get John to reveal his swimming cards. He'll never say how long we're going to be in the water for, however hard I attempt to wheedle it out of him.

An hour later, when we convene on the terrace for our daily briefing, he says that we're going out in a boat. He points to the edge of the headland, which marks the furthest point of land we can see from the house, and says we're going to go out there and swim home. He also says that we're going to practise feeding on the way back. Despite my love of food, eating in the ocean is not something I particularly fancy the thought of. But that's another thing I've learned about swimming the Channel – you don't do it without some form of sustenance on the way. Captain Matthew Webb drank beef tea and brandy in the nineteenth century, but fashions change and nowadays it's carbohydrate powder mixed with warm water and sweetened with fruit squash. John starts to give instructions about how it's going to be administered, how we need to drink it quickly so we don't stop for too long and get cold, and, most importantly, how we mustn't touch the boat during the process because if you do this during a Channel swim you'll be disqualified. But I'm not listening. All I can think about is how far that headland looks and how there's nearly no way I'm going to make it.

We jump on the boat from the water's edge and start to speed out to sea. It's only then that John discloses he's going to drop us all off the boat at different points. The strongest swimmers are going to be plopped in the water right at the headland and the aim is for them to swim and catch the rest of us up. A little closer to home he drops off a couple of others. And finally, but still along way out to sea, me.

John turns the boat to go back to check that the others are OK and suddenly I am alone, with only the deepest dark blue beneath me. It's a totally different experience from swimming up and down the shoreline. So far away from land, surrounded by water, I can sense the sea's immense power and its potential to extinguish human life in an instant. I also immediately imagine all the unknown, and possibly predatory, life forms around me and hope that whoever they are they'll stay away and let me share their world safely. But even though I feel small and vulnerable, as I start to swim I also feel something else. The words of a poem my dad used to recite to me when I was a child come unbidden into my mind: 'And truly I was afraid, I was most afraid, But even so, honoured still more.' As I swim I try to remember the rest of the poem and who wrote it but I find it impossible to focus on anything for very long as I'm constantly distracted by the effort of my movement through the water.

For what feels like ages I detect no sign of life or boat and I start to become more and more conscious of the cold. But I know now that minutes in water seem like hours and eventually, I hear the sound of the boat and John's voice.

'Hepburn, time for a feed,' he shouts.

I look up and see John leaning down with a cup. I reach up for it and take a sip. It is warm and sweet.

'Quickly,' he shouts. 'You don't want to get cold.'

'I already am,' I say.

'That's it, hand it back. Don't touch the boat,' he says, ignoring my comment.

I snatch another sip as John leans forward to take it and gives me my next instructions.

'Now start swimming. Quickly, so it gets into your bloodstream.'

I put my head down into the cold and for a few moments feel a glorious rush of warmth and energy. The boat speeds off and for a while I'm alone again, until suddenly I feel movement behind me. I flinch in fear before realising with relief it's just Andy and Mark, who have caught up with me.

For the rest of the way they swim alongside me. At first I think I'm doing a good job of keeping up with them, but it soon becomes clear they're just supporting and steering me home. As I swim, I think about the past week: how I've been a fish out of water – or should I say the only fish in the sea who doesn't like getting wet – but also how there has been something special about spending time in the company of strangers I would never usually meet in everyday life and doing something that I would never usually do. Here I am not 'Jessica the Infertile'; I am whoever I want to be – and although I wouldn't yet call myself 'Jessica the Swimmer', I do feel as if who I am is shifting a little.

Then, as I am thinking this, I suddenly remember the poem is by D. H. Lawrence. It's the one about his encounter with a snake. In it, he describes how he watches, mesmerised, as the snake drinks from his water trough and, despite the danger, and the voice of his education telling him to kill it, his first reaction is to feel honoured. And that's exactly how I'd felt, so far from land, in water so deep and unknown, because there is something exhilarating about surrendering yourself to an animal or element more powerful than you, especially when that thing – for me, the sea; for Lawrence, the snake – chooses to act kindly towards you. And as I swim into shore Lawrence's words rebound through the waves: 'Was it humility to feel so honoured?/ I felt so honoured . . .'*

---

* D. H. Lawrence, 'Snake', 1923

When we finally reach the beach, which looks near long before it is, the rest of the group are standing waiting.

'How was it?' they all say, 'or needn't we ask?!'

'Do you know what?' I reply. 'It was a tablespoon of agony and a teaspoon of amazing.'

Optimist or Pessimist?

'Helloooooooooooooooo,' the man in uniform calls.

I've got to the front of the passport queue and I didn't even realise it. For the last ten minutes I've been watching a woman and her daughter. The child – a toddler of around three or four – is wearing the cutest stripy OshKosh B'gosh dungarees and baseball boots. She's got her own miniature suitcase, fuchsia pink, which on her mother's instruction she picks up and carries forward each time the queue moves. I can't take my eyes off her. Occasionally, when she gets bored with the wait she abandons mother and suitcase and adventures under the barriers to explore, until her mum scoops her up and carries her back to the queue.

'Helloooooooooooooooo,' the man calls again.

I move towards the counter and hand over my passport, then head to the baggage carousel. I don't see her again.

Although it's already late afternoon when I get back, I have to head straight into work. It's the first day of rehearsals for a new production and in the evening we're having a party for all the actors and the staff to get to know each other. It begins with one of those games where everyone stands in a circle and reveals something unusual about themselves by way of introduction. Stupidly, when it's my turn, I say that I've just flown in from Spain where I've been training to swim the Channel. It's one of those moments when ego and adrenaline combine to make you say something you immediately regret. As soon as it's said, it can't be unsaid. For the rest of the evening people keep coming up to me and saying in admiration: 'Are you really?' I don't know how to answer this. If anything I'm even more unsure than I was before I went to Formentera. The week was good, but I didn't come anywhere close to doing six hours; even the headland swim was less than an hour and that felt like forever. A teaspoon of amazing doesn't get you from England to France.

The next day I get an email from John with an evaluation form. I hate evaluation forms. Whenever I get given one at a conference or event, it instantly becomes something to doodle on. I am a legendary doodler. Give me a piece of paper and a pen in a meeting and I won't write notes, but I will draw you lines of boxes and circles and stars. A stranger once leaned over to me and told me that my doodles said a lot about me. He left the meeting before it finished so I never got to ask him what they say exactly. Maybe they say, *I'm the type of woman who doesn't like filling out evaluation forms.* That would be true. However, I want to show my appreciation for the week away so I duly complete this one.

John emails me back:

> *Thanks Hepburn.*
>
> *Have you booked a boat yet for your Channel swim?*
>
> *To be so clear that you should after a week is not divine intervention in a prophetic vision that sees you successfully swim the Channel – it is an affirmation certainly from me to you that you have the potential which is a great start. As we discussed you would have to swim freestyle and to see you develop what is not your preferred stroke in such a short time was very encouraging. The encouragement is based upon your attitude and determination which as far as I know cannot be either filmed nor taught in a seminar. The opposing circumstance of a better stroke but flaws in both the mentioned characteristics would be a great cause for concern so you are on track ...*

In the days before the internet, this note would have arrived in the post and I would have let the ink fade and the paper go yellow and curl at the edges. It is a letter to treasure – so I print it out and pin it to the side of my desk. I certainly don't have a prophetic vision of me reaching the beach in France and picking up a pebble either, and I also know that attitude and determination doesn't get you everywhere, as otherwise I'd have a baby by now. But John's encouragement means a lot and I do have to think about what I'm going to do, because another thing I've learned is that swimming the Channel can never be a spur-of-the-moment decision. It involves months of planning and preparation.

The first thing you need to do is book a support boat. There are only a limited number registered to take people across in the small swimming window each summer. Over the next few days, I dare myself to look at the website, which has pictures of all the boats with their pilots. (I'm not sure why they're called pilots. I've always thought pilots flew planes and captains went to sea, which reminds me: flying is really a much better way of getting to France.) I clock a couple who look like they've got friendly faces and might be gentle on an amateur agonist. I email them to enquire about slots for next year. They seem to be very busy already but one, named Paul, has a slot on a neap tide next August.

Tides are another important factor in Channel swimming. There are two types, neaps and springs, and as far as I can tell, the main difference is that one has more water and is therefore stronger than the other. Historically, Channel soloists have always chosen to swim on the neaps, the one with less water, as it's considered to be easier.

Paul's boat is called *Optimist*, which seems like a good omen, but the problem is I've always been a pessimist and I can't bring myself to book it. To me, pessimism is the art of thinking that something won't happen so that when it doesn't you're not as disappointed as you might have been if you'd let yourself believe it would. I've found it to be the best protection from failure and disappointment and I've used it a lot over the last few years, as failure and disappointment seem to have been following me around. And the thing is, what if I'm just putting myself in their path again? It's all very well deciding to do something big, but I need it to be something I stand a chance of achieving.

Yet now I've thought it, how can I unthink it? I keep picturing myself at the end of my life with my bucket list in hand, recollecting that I wanted to be a mother (and wasn't), and that I wanted to swim the English Channel (and didn't even try). That feeling scares me, and over the next few days I've got Édith Piaf's 'Non, je ne regrette rien' playing on repeat in my head. But the pessimist in me still can't bring myself to book the *Optimist* because I'm even more terrified of facing failure and disappointment again.

A couple of days later I'm checking my work emails in bed before going to sleep. Apparently, this sort of thing kills your sex life, but then so does trying for a baby. No, that's not quite true. It's great when you start trying for a baby – there's nothing nicer than having sex for the purpose for which it was originally intended – what kills it is when you have to start trying very hard. I remember naively thinking that the first month we threw away that feminist-prized contraception, we'd be pregnant. But a month passed and nothing happened. Then two, then three, then more. We progressed to the ovulation predictor kit, designed to pinpoint the optimum moment for conception. But having sex to the tyranny of pee on a stick is a guaranteed passion-killer. It's now another of my 'nevers': never having sex for fun any more because sex is only about having a baby which never arrives.

Just before I close my laptop for the night, I decide to google and find out who the first woman to swim the Channel was. Everyone keeps talking about Captain Matthew Webb – the merchant seaman with the walrus moustache who was immortalised on a box of matches – but there must be a woman. I discover that she was an American named Gertrude Ederle. I laugh when I read that one of her most famous sayings was 'I eat whatever I want, whenever I want it.' She was definitely my kind of girl. So I get out my list of women who changed the world and add a special entry. Number twenty-one: Gertrude Ederle. Her position on the list seems serendipitous – the exact number of miles from England to France. She lived to the age of ninety-eight and it turns out she's another woman who never became a mother. I wonder why and whether the sea was her 'darling child'.

I put down my laptop and think about Ms Stiller's email. It was nice of her to reply when I wrote and she's right, of course: I'm never really going to know what Jane Austen, Gertrude Ederle or any of the women on my list truly thought about not having children. I'm never going to know how happy it made them that they did something big instead. Then I close my eyes and think about *Optimist*, the support boat available on the neap tide starting on 21 August next year. And then I think about the little girl with her pink suitcase and I wonder if that's a tide that can ever turn. And thinking all these things, I eventually fall asleep. But the next day, as soon as I wake up, I send an email to Paul the pilot to book his boat. I've had an idea about how swimming the Channel might help me decide what to do next in my pursuit of motherhood. Besides, I can always cancel the booking, if that baby does decide to arrive.

Half a Biscuit

BBC Radio 4 is coming over to interview me about my IVF story. This is a major moment. Seeing my legs in the most read tabloid newspaper in the world is nothing compared to hearing my voice on Radio 4. I love Radio 4. I have done since I was at university and a boy I had a crush on persuaded me to start listening to it. The crush was unrequited, but a lifelong radio love affair began. I just wish I hadn't had to fail at having a baby in order to succeed at being on it. But putting that aside, it's Radio 4. RADIO 4!!!

Now, I've been asked to be part of a documentary which is going to be written and presented by a BBC journalist who has decided to come out for the first time about her own struggle to conceive. The producer calls and says they want to do at least part of the interview with me at home. Apparently background sound is very important in radio as it adds colour. They want to record me boiling the kettle, that kind of stuff. I'm not sure how I feel about this. If I'm honest I don't really want them to come round. Not just because I'll have to tidy up but also because it feels like a further 'opening-up' of our life that I'm not sure even I'm comfortable with.

A few days later, hesitation cast recklessly aside, the producer and presenter arrive. The presenter is petite, pretty and clearly clever. We stand together talking in the kitchen whilst I put the coffee on – one of those silver stovetop pots that heat up on the hob. The producer points her furry microphone towards it. As the water comes to the boil it makes a satisfying bubbly sound. The producer moves the microphone closer. We carry on talking. I offer to warm some milk. It boils over, white foam cascading over the top of the saucepan. Embarrassed, I take out mugs from the cupboard. Huge ones – the size of bowls – decorated with beautiful multicoloured streams of paint that looks like it's running off an easel. I like them a lot. They're my best mugs. I pour out the coffee. It looks a bit weak. Then I pour over the burned milk. It curdles.

This isn't going well. I want to come across as someone who is confident with people in the kitchen. I have always dreamed of living in a country farmhouse: a well-used wooden table on a flagstone floor surrounded by family; bread and cakes cooling on wire racks; homemade jams and pickles in Le Parfait jars. The sort of place where there would always be people talking, laughing, eating and drinking and I would be mother-cum-maître d'. Instead we live in a shoebox in central London which is so small we rarely have people round. We don't have a table to speak of and, it seems, I've even lost the skill to make a visitor a cup of coffee. How is it that my life is so far away from the dreams I had? There's nothing to stop me living in a farmhouse. I could still make cakes and jam. But I don't, and there is something about where we've chosen to live that I know is a by-product of our childlessness.

We sit down. The presenter is on a chair, balancing the cup, which is almost as big as her, on her knees. She doesn't look comfortable; I'm not comfortable. It makes me wonder why I'm putting us all through this. Then I remember the biscuits.

'I bought biscuits,' I say, jumping up excitedly and nearly knocking over my own cup. 'Two packs. Posh ones – pistachio or sultana. Which would you prefer?'

The presenter and the producer both make mmm-ing sounds but don't give me a definitive answer, so I open both packets and put a few of each in a bowl. The producer takes one. The presenter politely refuses. She doesn't look like the sort of woman who eats a lot of biscuits. I decide not to have one either.

And so the interview starts. Here we go again. Infertility. IVF. The sadness. The shame. The envy. The emptiness. At one point the presenter cries, and then shares a little of her own story. She's Asian and I had wondered if this might have its own particular challenges. She tells me it does, that in traditional Asian communities, couples without children are shunned and women are often the ones who are blamed. And then she suddenly takes a biscuit, breaks it carefully in half, puts one half down and starts eating the other.

After two hours of conversation, the producer thanks me. She says we've generated some great material but she's wondering whether there's anywhere else they could record me – ideally with interesting background noise?

'Somewhere else?' I say, half in question, half in astonishment that two hours of intimate disclosure in my kitchen and a bubbling coffee pot hasn't been enough.

'Have you got any friends or family that are having a children's party in the next few weeks?' she asks. 'That might work well.'

'Not that I can think of,' I say. (Knowing I can't think of anything worse.)

'Or do you have any particular hobbies or places that you like to go that have a good soundscape?'

'Well, there is somewhere,' I say, desperate to respond with an alternative to the humiliation of a children's party. 'I've started swimming at the Serpentine in Hyde Park some mornings. It's got ducks – could be good for radio?'

'Yes . . . that could work,' the producer ponders.

'So you're a swimmer?' the presenter asks.

'Not exactly,' I reply. 'Although I do have this crazy idea that I want to try and swim the English Channel next year.'

'Wow,' the presenter and the producer say in unison.

We then have the no-wetsuit and it's-going-to-take-at-least-fifteen-hours conversation.

'Wow,' they both say again.

'So is this about you trying to move on?' the presenter asks.

I notice that something inside me feels immediately defensive and, as if she senses that she's pressed a bruise, she doesn't wait for my answer and says instead: 'Are you doing it for charity?'

Ever since I publicly announced my Channel aspirations at work, people have been asking this question, and I haven't had an answer. What am I doing it for? I realise I lied to my colleagues when I said I'd never done a sponsored anything before. I did a sponsored walk once, when I was at primary school, and raised about 20p. I had been hopeless at asking people for money. So I sidestep this question too by saying I haven't decided yet but that I do have another idea.

'Yes?' the presenter says looking interested.

'To be honest, I haven't told anyone yet but maybe I could try it out on you and see what you think?'

This is the first time I've spoken aloud the idea that came to me the night I decided to book my boat, but now another thought has occurred to me about how the presenter might be able to help.

'Sure,' she replies.

'Well, because of the cold and the no-wetsuit rule, you have to put on weight to swim the Channel.'

'Yes . . .'

'So I thought I might write to some inspirational women – some of them mothers, some of them not – and ask them to meet and eat with me. I thought I could ask them whether they think motherhood makes you happy or whether you can have a fulfilling life without children. It might help me decide what to do next in my own pursuit of motherhood.'

'Sounds great,' the presenter says encouragingly. 'You should.'

I pause for a moment, summoning bravery.

'Actually, I was just wondering, and I hope you don't

mind me asking ... but I'm wondering ...' I take a breath and press on nervously. 'I'm wondering whether I could interview *you* over lunch or dinner or something?'

'Interview *me*?' the presenter says.

She looks startled and I immediately fear I've gone too far. She pauses before speaking again – presumably to work out how to let me down tactfully – so I step in and save her. 'Don't worry, you don't need to say yes now. Have a think about it. I'll write to you another time,' I say, speaking quickly to cover all our embarrassment, 'or maybe I could just have the transcript of our conversation today?' I add, turning to the producer and then back to the presenter. 'I know we didn't eat but I did make you a coffee which you've been so nice about drinking even though I burned the milk. And you had a biscuit. Well – half a biscuit.'

Oh God, I think, I shouldn't have mentioned the biscuit. Now I've made things even worse.

The presenter smiles at me kindly without really giving an answer. The producer, who I can tell doesn't want to do anything without the presenter's agreement, says she'll ask her boss about the transcript. I don't push it. I move on. We all know she's not going to ask her boss about the transcript. Maybe it was naive of me to think that anyone in the public eye would be prepared to talk to me candidly about their thoughts on motherhood versus non-motherhood, especially a journalist who, after all, is accustomed to being the interviewer not interviewee.

As I show them out, the producer says she'll be in touch about recording me at the Serpentine. I feel a knot of regret in my stomach. Why did I mention any of that swimming stuff? What was I thinking when I booked that boat? None of this is going to get me what I really want.

———

Later that evening, I decide it's got to be beer and nachos for supper. Sometimes the only thing that helps is a jalapeño.

The Serpentine

The Serpentine Swimming Club in London's Hyde Park is one of the most legendary open-water swimming clubs in the world. It has probably nurtured more Channel swimmers than any other club in England and given that it's the nearest natural swimming location to where we live it was probably inevitable that I would find my way there. I say natural, but actually the Serpentine lake was created at the request of Queen Caroline, wife of George II, in 1730. (Going back to my list of women who changed the world that's after Elizabeth I and before Victoria.) For centuries Hyde Park had been a royal hunting ground, until Charles I opened it to the public in 1637. Around a hundred years later, Caroline decided she wanted to create an ornamental lake to make the park even more beautiful. At the time most artificial lakes were long and straight but the Serpentine, which was named for its snake-like shape, was one of the first man-made lakes to curve as if it was natural.

The first time I ventured down was a cold, wet, winter morning at the start of my Channel exploration – around about the time I made my first call to John. I'd read that the club – situated at the bit of the lake known as the Serpentine Lido, which has been roped off to create a swimming enclosure of a hundred metres in length – was a good place to meet people who had swum the Channel. So I decided to go on a reconnaissance mission. I'd also read that the best time to meet them was at the famous Saturday morning races – which have been running for well over a hundred years and take place every week, year round – when swimmers compete over various distances for a series of different cups linked to figures associated with the club's history.

When I arrived the banks of the lake near the lido were crowded with people and it was difficult to work out quite what was going on. A group of swimmers, clad only in swimming costumes and silicon hats, were lining up along the pontoon jutting out into the water at one end of the lido. Then a man on the edge – clothed much more appropriately for a winter's morning – started counting through a microphone and one by one at intermittent intervals each member of the group descended into the murky, chilly-looking water and started swimming. Any stroke seemed to go – crawl, breaststroke; there was even a butterflyer. Eventually they were all in and swimming at full pelt up towards the top of the roped-off enclosure where they got out. Then the whole thing started again with a new batch of swimmers. The juxtaposition of near-naked bodies jumping into the cold with people standing on the bank wrapped up in coats and hats was an incongruous one. I watched for a while and then at what I hoped was an opportune moment sidled over to the man with the microphone and asked if he knew whether there was anyone around who had swum the Channel.

'Go and speak to Boris and Nick,' he said, pointing towards two men standing a short distance away, both over six feet tall, mid-thirties-ish, and embodying the word 'strapping'. I introduced myself. They were polite and told me where to look for more information on the internet, but there was nothing about our conversation on that Saturday morning that made me feel encouraged to believe I could do what they had done. If anything, it made me think that this was a closed world I didn't belong in. However, what I realise now is that no one who has swum the English Channel, or knows anything about Channel swimming, will tell a stranger in a gung-ho fashion that they can definitely do it. Because you can't. Even the strongest swimmers rule themselves out of the Everest of swimming. And these men didn't know me from Poseidon.

I didn't attempt a swim that morning. After my conversation I sloped off for breakfast at the café overlooking the east side of the lake. But I did think to myself that eggs Benedict might taste even nicer if you'd been in the water, and figured that at least thinking that was a move in the right direction.

———

The next time I ventured down to the Serpentine was the Saturday after I got back from Formentera. Andy, Mark and Teresa were all members of the club and with their encouragement I decided to give it another go. It helped that it was now mid-April and the weather and water were getting warmer. Still cold, though. Very cold. They had also helpfully explained the whole counting thing to me, which is to do with a handicap system that ensures everyone has an equal chance of winning the race whatever stroke or speed they swim at. What happens is that you are a given a number on which you start the race, which is gradually refined over time as week by week the club's Honorary Handicapper gets to know your speed. The slowest swimmers have the lowest numbers and go off first, while the faster ones have higher numbers and chase after them.

The morning of my second visit to the Serpentine, the race involved everyone swimming from the pontoon to the top of the lido enclosure, back again, then down to a buoy about the same distance away on the other side and finally returning to the pontoon, a total distance of 400 metres. I got given a handicap and my heart was beating fast as I heard the number approaching. When it arrived there seemed little choice but to get in. The thrashing of bodies all around me in cold water was overwhelming. Handicap or no handicap, I didn't win.

That morning, in addition to my baptism, I also had my initiation into the Serpentine's spartan changing facilities: one small room with wooden benches and hooks on three sides, a sink in the corner and an adjoining toilet. There's no segregation between men and women; everyone just crowds in and you quickly get used to the odd flash of breast or buttock. The only nod to modern times is one of those clever machines hanging over the sink that supplies instant hot water to ensure that tea is on tap. There's also a regular supply of biscuits and cakes (often homemade) brought in to share with fellow swimmers. Or should I say fellow eccentrics. Because the members of the Serpentine Swimming Club are a raggle-taggle bunch. From impoverished artists to merchant millionaires; from teenagers to octogenarians; from those who were born to the sound of Bow Bells to those who were educated at Eton: all united by a love of swimming in the open air.

And since then I've been returning. Mostly reluctantly, because there is nothing about the exercise or the cold water that is getting easier, even as the months are getting warmer. But I do quite enjoy the walk through Hyde Park and saying to the ducks, 'Hello, here I am again, dreading it as usual!' And, just as I did in Formentera, I am staying in slightly longer each time, and when I get out covered in green slime I notice Boris and Nick looking at me approvingly, and that feels good. I'm still a novice, but when I reluctantly concede to the BBC Radio 4 team recording me there, I do a pretty good job of looking like I know the protocol. But there's a world of difference between a lap of the lake and swimming the Channel. Me and the ducks both know that.

Does Motherhood Make You Happy?

Today I discovered an interesting piece of Serpentine trivia. On Tuesday 10 December 1816, a heavily pregnant woman was found drowned in the middle of the lake. She left a suicide note addressed to her father, sister and husband. Her name was Harriet Westbrook and she was the wife of the Romantic poet Percy Bysshe Shelley. Just two weeks after her death, Shelley married again – some people might consider this to be in unseemly haste. His new bride was a young woman called Mary, who happened to be the daughter of Mary Wollstonecraft, one of my original twenty women (now twenty-one). After the marriage she became Mary Shelley, and but for Sappho, Virginia Woolf and Jane Austen, she might have made the list herself as the author of *Frankenstein*, one of the greatest Gothic novels of all time. The Shelleys – Mary and Percy – were very much in love, and lost three children in pregnancy before finally having a son. Water was then to play a part in their fate again when Percy drowned off the coast of Italy. Mary was only twenty-five at the time and never remarried. So it just goes to show, even if you do something big in your life, even if it's big enough to always be remembered, you could still be only a stroke away from tragedy. And that's why you can't let the small disappointments in life hold you back. The presenter wasn't going to work out, but I can't let that stop me. I decide it's time to start another list.

―――――――――

I open my laptop and at the top of the page I type the heading 'Mothers'. I then tab down about half a screen of white space and write 'Non-Mothers'.

Starting with the 'Mothers' section, I mentally mull through all the living people I can think of who are well known for motherhood. I type: 'the Queen' – she is, after all, the matriarchal head of the most famous family in Britain. But it's undoubtedly a long shot. Then underneath I write: 'Katie Price', followed by 'Kerry Katona'. With ten children between them and careers built largely on magazine features and reality television programmes about them, their ever-changing husbands and their children, both women have made being a mother a professional occupation. Another long shot, I guess, unless either *OK!* magazine or I are prepared to pay.

Next I scroll down to the 'Non-Mothers' section, think for a moment and then type 'Jennifer Aniston'. Is there anyone else in the world who has had to endure more conjecture about whether or not she's pregnant or wants to become a mother? Her situation has not been helped by the fact that for years she was cast in the role of tragic heroine as a result of her ex-husband Brad Pitt's relationship with Angelina Jolie. I scroll back up to 'Mothers' and type 'Angelina Jolie', and then I create a new subsection called 'Adoptive Mothers' and write her name again. With a total of six children – three adopted, three biological – Jolie has to be one of the most extraordinary combinations of mother, Hollywood star and humanitarian campaigner the world has ever seen, only really rivalled by Audrey Hepburn before her. If Angelina or Audrey decided they wanted to swim the Channel for charity, they're the kind of women who probably wouldn't even need to get wet.

Over the course of the next few weeks the list grows. New subsections emerge under the overarching title of 'Mothers' in order to differentiate the various routes that women have taken to achieve this status. As well as 'Adoptive Mothers' I add 'Foster Mothers', and if people have been public about having to use assisted conception I put them under headings entitled 'IVF', 'Surrogacy' and 'Egg Donation'. It's harder to categorise the 'Non-Mothers', but there are subsections here too. There are those women who never wanted to become mothers and are child-free by choice. And there are the women who did want to become mothers, but because of a variety of circumstances have not done so. It's quite hard to decipher which is which. Of course, ultimately, every woman in the world could be on my list. They're in one category or another. But as I add people, I find myself drawn to those who have an interesting story to tell around being or not being a mother. Some are household names, others are famous in their particular field, and others are women who very few people may have heard of but who have done something quietly amazing.

For quite a long time it's just me and the list and nobody knows. It gets longer and longer: there's no way I'm going to be able to meet and eat with everyone on it. But that's OK. I can't imagine the Queen will say yes. Or Jennifer Aniston and Angelina Jolie for that matter. But ultimately if a plan is going to come to fruition, dreaming doesn't do it. Something has to happen to force the movement of thought into action.

And then it does. Someone posts a message on one of the Channel swimming internet forums saying they have to cancel their swim this coming August and offering up their slot if anyone wants to take it. If I could get a team together, it would be a chance to do a relay which, as John has said, would be a good way of seeing what swimming the Channel is really like.

I take it and the next day, emboldened by a full English breakfast after a swim in the Serpentine, I start composing my letters, determined to keep writing until someone eventually says 'yes':

> *Dear . . . [fill in name here]*
> *I am writing to ask whether you would meet and eat with me to help me get fat to swim the English Channel and answer the question: Does motherhood make you happy?*

The Etiquette of Clothing

Spend any significant length of time with open-water swimmers and you'll soon learn that the etiquette of clothing is very important. I had quickly established that you can't wear a wetsuit if you want to be classified as a Channel swimmer, but in fact they are anathematised in general. Read this from the Serpentine rulebook:

> Concerning wetsuits, we recognise that some external events are 'wetsuit-compulsory' and people need to use them for training. However, their use is considered by many not to be within the true spirit of an all year round open-air swimming club.

The true spirit of the Serpentine is skins. Thankfully, this isn't quite what it sounds. You don't have to risk arrest for indecent exposure in Hyde Park. You can wear a swimming costume. But there are also pretty strict rules in open-water swimming on what constitutes a costume. It should be of a material not offering any form of thermal protection or buoyancy. It should be sleeveless (i.e. no creep below the shoulders) and legless (i.e. nothing that extends to the upper leg below the crotch). You can wear a hat. Hats are legit as long as you only wear one of them. But don't even begin to think about those nifty boots or gloves. Covering your hands and feet is strictly prohibited. Goose fat, whilst allowed, has long gone out of fashion. Contrary to what people used to think, it doesn't keep you warm, it just makes you sticky, and it's impossible to get off. But for long swims it is advisable to rub a bit of grease in places prone to chafing. That was one of the things I learned in Formentera, where some of the customs of this strange world had been revealed to me for the first time.

But the etiquette of clothing doesn't end there. It's not just about what you wear in the water, it's also about what you put on afterwards. You have approximately ten minutes after getting out of the water before the afterdrop occurs, more commonly known as 'the shivers'. Use that time wisely and get dressed as quickly as possible. Replace your swimming hat with a woolly version, even if it's a bright sunny day. Take off your costume and put on warm clothes. And my top tip is: go commando. There is nothing more fiddly than a bra and knickers when you're cold, so go without – with all the layers nobody's going to know.

I have also recently discovered a fabulous accoutrement called the Dryrobe. The clue is in the title: a robe that keeps you dry. It's a huge, hooded black cloak which makes you look a bit like the Grim Reaper. If you put it on as soon as you leave the water, you can get changed under it and then huddle in it to get warm. I can tell that all the hardcore open-water swimmers are a bit disdainful of the Dryrobe. Boris and Nick don't have one. My hunch is that it's not because of the way it looks but because it offers a bit too much comfort for the elite cold-water athlete. But even those who do own one – and there are lots who do – seem to shed it before encountering civilisation. Not me. I wear mine home on the tube. Everyone at the Serpentine thinks this is hysterical but I don't understand what's funny. Just call me Jessica, the Grim Reaper.

And finally, there's one more piece of clothing that has also changed my life since I started swimming in the open air. Shoelaces. Not the ones that are impossible to tie up when your fingers are shaking with the cold but the fizzy strawberry liquorice ones. They are manna after a swim. Whoever decided to turn laces into liquorice was a genius. Swimming and woolly hats off to him.

The Charity Worker

'The important thing is you live your life authentically.'

I love Waterloo Bridge. But not when it's raining.

I looked out of the window this morning and there was a fine sheet of drizzle, which I chose to ignore. I'd already decided what I was going to wear: my light blue summer dress with my bright blue-and-green silk scarf. I didn't have an alternative. The scarf is the most vibrant thing in my wardrobe and the first woman who had agreed to meet me and talk about motherhood is someone I wanted to honour with colour – the etiquette of clothing is very important to her too. But the main problem was my shoes. The only ones I've got that go with the outfit are a pair of cheap ballet pumps, and by the time I've left our flat and walked the short distance to Waterloo Bridge, they have virtually disintegrated in the rain – that will teach me for buying £7 shoes which have probably been made in some terrible sweatshop.

The cupcakes I've bought are suffering too. I'd spent a long time thinking about what to bring. She had invited me to her office at noon but there'd been no mention of food in the email. Although noon is bordering on lunchtime, I didn't want to be presumptuous, so I'd decided to bring a selection of colourful cakes. I'd spent a long time choosing them. The shop assistant had been very patient with me as I tried out various colour combinations. In the end I settled on light pink, dark pink, blue, yellow, cream and brown. But by the time I am halfway across the bridge, the large paper bag they are in has become sodden, the handle has broken and, even worse, the cakes in their beautiful box have collapsed into one another and are a multicoloured mess.

The person I have come to meet and (hopefully) eat cake with is Camila Batmanghelidjh, who founded the charity Kids Company (although a year after we meet it would close down[2]). She is as well known for her sartorial splendour as she is for her outspoken views on the plight of disadvantaged young people. But the thing that has always fascinated me about Camila is that, despite her obvious love of children, she has never had any herself. In fact, she has often been quoted in newspaper articles as saying she never had any desire to become a mother. I wanted to find out whether this was true and to see if it's possible for someone to be a mother without being a mother. I was thrilled when she replied to my letter and agreed to see me.

When I arrive at her office in Southwark, just south of the Thames, I have to wait for a while because Camila has been called to help with an incident concerning a young person and the police. Her staff tell me that the girl involved won't talk to the authorities unless Camila is there. The children and teenagers she works with clearly trust her.

After about ten minutes, she appears.

Camila Batmanghelidjh is one of those people whose presence in a room is impossible to ignore – partly because she is physically imposing, partly because of her flamboyant robes and turban, and partly because she has just that, a presence. She shakes my hand warmly and leads me into her office, which is unlike any office I have ever been in. It is large and dimly lit, with a collection of elaborate lampshades hanging over a round table in one corner and a circle of armchairs in another. The floor is covered in ethnic rugs; the walls are filled floor to ceiling with children's pictures. It's such an assault on the senses that it's impossible to take it all in with one sweep of the eyes. Suffice to say, the girl who was raised in Iran until the revolution has made sure that if the sultans of Persia ever come to visit they're sure to feel at home. As for the children from the streets of London, well, they probably think they're in a scene from Disney's *Aladdin*.

I take out the box of cakes, apologising for the rain damage and assuring her that she doesn't need to eat one.

'Don't worry,' she laughs, taking them from me. 'Would *you* like one?'

'Well, I had rather set my heart on that one,' I say, pointing to the one covered in cream icing and a sprinkling of hundreds-and-thousands which now also has a streak of cerise pink on one side and aquamarine blue on the other. Camila lifts the cake out of the box, hands it to me across the table and then conjures a pair of plastic teaspoons from somewhere. She takes out a cake for herself and scoops off a bit of the icing, avoiding the sponge. That's all she eats. One teaspoonful. Maybe two. I, on the other hand, decide to use my spoon as a knife, cutting my cake into quarters and devouring all four. I'm not the sort of girl who eats cake with a teaspoon: you can't get enough purchase on the sponge.

I take out my laptop and place it on the table with my list of questions in front of me. I'm nervous – I'm not a journalist. It's the first time I've done anything like this. I'm also conscious that I haven't got long with her, so I hurtle in headlong, saying that although I know she made the decision not to have children early on in her life, I'd like to know whether she ever considered having them. She says she didn't and that she has never regretted it, which, given her love of children, she realises is strange. So I ask how she decided what she wanted to do with her life.

'It had no option,' she replies instantly. 'It was so powerful. Even as a young child I had an intuition about doing something for which I had no vocabulary. I remember thinking that I needed the words to describe this thing that I knew.'

I'm struck by the fact that she refers to her life in the third person, as if it is somehow separate from her, and I ask whether she thinks some of the most iconic maternal figures who didn't have children – such as Mother Teresa and Florence Nightingale (both on my list of women who changed the world) – might have felt the same.

'I don't know,' she says, 'but what I have thought is that Western psychology is a bit limited on this subject. It's so focused around the idea of personal need. But maybe there's another type of psyche which we haven't got round to describing yet, which is much less interested in individual fulfilment and more driven by vocation, public duty, the psychology of compassion.'

'So what if you want to become a mother *and* you want to do something bigger with your life?' I ask. 'Can you have a psyche in conflict?'

She looks at me knowingly and smiles. 'Yes, you can have a conflict,' she says, 'but the fact that you are experiencing one, Jessica, suggests your own personal life drive is more dominant.'

I'm embarrassed that she has immediately recognised I am talking about myself.

'And there's nothing wrong with that,' Camila adds quickly. 'Neither is good or bad, and wanting to be a mother doesn't stop you from being creative. But there's a difference between a creative life and a vocational life. A vocational life means living that vocation 100 per cent. It sounds to me like what you want is motherhood with a creative outlet. So just be honest with yourself and say, "That's what I want," and live it. The important thing is you live your life authentically.'

'But what if you can't become a mother? I mean biologically. Do you think you can become a mother in other ways?' I ask.

'I do, although I do think it goes in grades. People who have given birth to their own child have a bond that is very deep and instinctual, even if it's through a donor. Then the next level is adopting a child as a baby or through a surrogate. Again that bond is deep because you are growing the child from the beginning, but it won't be quite as profound. And then you go a bit further up if you adopt a child that is slightly older. I know I have a deep love for the children I care for even though not a single one belongs to me, but I am also realistic that there is an intrinsic attachment that I don't have because I never gave birth to them.'

'And do they love you?'

'They love me deeply but they love their biological carer more – however abusive that relationship is. The truth is that if you take another route you will have to accept that there will always be a third mother in the relationship.'

'I'm not sure how *my* psyche will cope with that.'

'You just need to acknowledge that the relationship exists. Things go wrong when people pretend otherwise. But you do have to accept there will be times when your child will absolutely despise you and have fantasies that this other mother will be better.'

I admit to her that I'm more worried about my own fantasies: the ones telling me that I'm not supposed to be a mother and that the third mother *will* be better. She looks at me, a look that penetrates my core.

'Jessica, I think there is something important for you to gain from this journey you've set out on, which is meeting your truth. You can cope with anything provided you have faced the truth of it. It all goes wrong when people engage in emotional pretences. So visit it now and then make your decision.'

A moment's silence falls between us as we both contemplate the veracity of what she's just said. I glance over at the questions on my laptop and notice my time with her is running out.

'What makes you happy?' I ask.

Her eyes start to sparkle. 'Being in water,' she says. 'I just love being in water.'

'Really? You like swimming?' I say. This is an unexpected revelation.

'I've always loved it,' she replies. 'Since I was a child and I went swimming in the Caspian Sea. I swim for four, five, six hours at a time.'

'Wow! You could swim the Channel!' I say.

'I could,' she says confidently. 'Yeah, I could swim the Channel.' And then she tells me that she was born very prematurely and she thinks there's something driving her back to fluids. Sadly, I don't think there's anything driving me back to fluids; if anything, something keeps pushing me away. When I say this she laughs, and I wonder what she must think of me – the woman with the psyche that doesn't really know what it wants, the swimmer who doesn't really want to swim.

'I have one last question,' I say as I close my laptop.

'Yes?'

'I'm going to ask it of every woman who agrees to meet and eat with me, and given your love of swimming you're the perfect person to start with.'

'Yes?'

'Well, the swim is going to take many hours so I need to find something to do to pass the time. Will you give me a word to motivate me to keep swimming that I can recite to myself?' I ask. 'One word. Any word,' I say, waiting for her to think.

'"Delicious",' she says suddenly, savouring the word as she says it. 'The water is delicious, so don't fight it.'

The Scientist

'Doing something hard and achieving it . . .
that's what real happiness is.'

How do you address a professor who is also a baroness: Professor? Baroness? Professor Baroness? Baroness Professor?

Or just Susan?

Susan Greenfield is a scientist. A professor of neuroscience, to be precise. And in 2001 she was awarded a life peerage and became a baroness. She's not a mother and has said in the past that it's very difficult to achieve a successful scientific career if you're a woman who has children. This is not strictly true, of course: Marie Curie, number nineteen on my list and the first woman to win a Nobel Prize for science (in fact she won two, one in 1903 for physics, one in 1911 for chemistry), had two children, but it's an interesting and important statement nonetheless. I want to know more about why Susan Greenfield had decided not to have them and whether she is happy.

I write to her via her website and within a few hours get an email back from her PA saying that Baroness Greenfield (so there's my answer) is too busy to meet and eat at the moment but she could give me fifteen minutes on the phone next Tuesday morning at ten. I accept, despite the fact that I'm supposed to be in an important meeting which starts at half-past nine. I've decided that my policy is: if I get offered a day and time, I've got to take it; she who hesitates and all that. It's kind of how I feel about the Channel. If I hesitate, it ain't happening.

When the day comes, I arrive early for my work meeting to finesse the details of my fifteen-minute absence from it midway through. The woman who's hosting kindly offers me her office to take the call. I don't say what it's about and thankfully she doesn't ask. I'm not quite sure how I'd explain that I'm interviewing one of the country's top scientists, on work time, about what it feels like not to be a mother.

I'd purposefully skipped breakfast, assuming that as the work meeting was starting early there'd be something laid on. I figured that even if the baroness wasn't eating, I could have coffee and a pastry while talking to her. But there are only some pale-looking custard creams laid out on the table and, frankly, biscuits do not a breakfast make. Just before ten, I pour myself a cup of black coffee and leave the room.

There is an oversized clock on the wall in the office I'm borrowing and I sit waiting for the hands to reach the allotted time. I'm nervous. The moment they hit ten, I pick up the phone and dial the number. It rings once before she answers.

'Is that Baroness Greenfield?' I say.

A voice at the end of the line says, 'Jessica?'

'It's Jessica Hepburn,' I reply and then feel immediately

stupid. She knows it's me, that's why she just said my name. I fumble on, thanking her for agreeing to speak to me and acknowledging that I've been told she doesn't have long to talk.

'About ten minutes?' she says briskly.

I decide it would be churlish to remark that her PA had actually offered me fifteen and say instead that I've got a few questions, apologising if they're a bit 'deep' for first thing on a Tuesday morning.

'That's OK,' she says, her voice softening slightly. 'Off you go.'

I ask my first question – what did she want to be when she grew up? – and she says that's easy: she wanted to be a horse-riding instructor because she was mad about ponies and used go riding every weekend. Maybe not the most obvious hobby for a working-class girl from London. But then again, I don't suppose anyone would have expected her to become a world expert on the brain either.

I want to know more but I'm two minutes down and have to move on, so next I ask whether motherhood ever figured, hoping she won't find the question too intrusive. She doesn't seem to and tells me that up until she was thirteen she was an only child, but then her little brother was born. She says the shock and squalor of having a baby in the house screaming and soiling his nappies made motherhood seem very unpalatable. Then, when she grew up, she became so deeply involved with and fulfilled by her work that it was hard to reconcile it with the thought of becoming a mother. And, finally, she got married aged forty to a man who already had a daughter and made it clear he didn't want any more children.

She speaks quickly, like people with big brains often do. But having said all this she pauses for a moment and then says more slowly: 'I suppose you could say it was a combination of non-game-changing factors that ended up changing the game. If I'd known I really wanted to become a mother maybe things might have been different, but I was never sure and it never happened.'

'That's a great line,' I say, trying to furiously scribble down everything she's said.

'What?'

'A combination of non-game-changing factors that ended up changing the game . . . kind of like life.'

'Yes,' she agrees, and although I can't see her, I think I can feel her smile.

I want to ask her more about motherhood but she's done such a good job of explaining why it didn't happen and seems so relaxed about the way the game of her life has played out that it doesn't seem appropriate.

'What's happiness to you?' I say instead.

'Doing something hard and achieving it. You know, like proving a scientific theory. I enjoy dancing and drinking and those sorts of things but doing something hard and achieving it, that's what real happiness is.'

I think about the 'hardness' of the Channel.

'And how would you like to be remembered?' I say.

'Oh, that's easy,' she says quickly. 'For finding a cure to Alzheimer's.'

I'm not quite sure how to respond to this. My knowledge of how the cure for Alzheimer's is progressing is not good. 'So . . . how's it . . . going then?' I say tentatively, hoping it's not too stupid a question.

'Well, we're making progress,' she answers and then her voice turns swift and sharp. 'But we're not there yet. So don't say that I said we are, because we're not.'

Maybe she's not there yet, but I can't help thinking that Alzheimer's research is in capable hands. If I were going to put my money on anyone finding a cure, then I'd bet on the baroness. I kind of wish she'd chosen to focus on dysfunctional wombs rather than the brain.

I'm conscious that my time is running out and if I want to ask her more about the subject of motherhood, I'd better get on with it, so I apologise for my next question, saying that I know she's already explained why she didn't become a mother, but does she think that motherhood is important in the fulfilment of a woman's life?

'Well, this seems like a simplistic answer,' she says matter-of-factly, 'but for women for whom it's important, it's important.'

I now definitely feel stupid. It's not a simplistic answer, it's a simplistic bloody question. But instead of waiting for me to find a better next question, she continues talking: 'It saddens me that some women are pressurised culturally to feel that they need to have a child. And that many women who don't or can't are regarded as objects of pity and feel they have to justify it in some way because somehow it's unnatural or abnormal.' There is a sudden urgency in her voice as she says this, as if it's something she feels strongly about. 'I object to the fact that men don't feel stigmatised in the same way. It just isn't an issue whether they have children or not and they wouldn't dream of discussing it, but whenever I meet another woman who hasn't had children, I still feel like I have to say, "Neither do I", as if somehow it's important to share our difference.'

As she says this I realise that here is a woman who has felt the stigma of not being a mother even if she's not felt the pain, and that although these feelings are very different they are also somehow the same. Because we are still living in a world where even being a top scientist who might one day find the cure for Alzheimer's is not enough to surpass society's expectations that women ought to be mothers and if they're not there's something wrong with them. Who asked Darwin whether he was a dad? Probably no one. (He was. He had ten children. Not even Marie Curie could manage that.)

'I know you've got to go but I just have one last question if I may?'

'Yes?'

I ask her for one word. She hesitates for a moment, as if she doesn't quite understand.

'It could be one that you particularly like, or something to inspire me,' I say.

'"Life",' she says suddenly and defiantly. 'My word for you is life.'

So the baroness gives me life, but I can't help thinking that what's far more important is the life she's working so hard to give other people. And as I put down the phone the thought that absorbs me more than anything is that the most significant thing this woman can achieve in this world is not to be a mother, but for her wish of how she'll be remembered to come true.

The Old Woman of Coniston

I blame Chris for Lake Coniston. I haven't introduced you to Chris yet. In fact, I wasn't sure I was going to. I met him in Formentera with the others, where he was the one and only person to do his six-hour qualifier for his Channel solo this summer. He's a good swimmer and a nice guy but he's one of my doubters. Boris and Nick from the Serpentine are doubters too. They haven't said it but I know they are. John, for all his encouragement, may also be a doubter and is just keeping it to himself. But Chris, well, Chris is an official doubter. When he found out I'd booked my Channel swim for the following year, he told me outright I didn't stand a chance unless I was prepared to start swimming seriously. Seriously is a euphemism for faster, longer and better. He said that as well as doing a Channel relay this summer I should attempt Coniston in the Lake District to see how I get on.

At just over five miles long Coniston is a quarter of the width of the Channel, but without the tides taking you all over the place. And the jellyfish, of course. It will be the biggest swim I've ever attempted, but it's time to take the doubters on.

Each year, there are several organised swims of the lake between July and September when the water's at its warmest, although many people still choose to swim it in a wetsuit. We arrive late at night, the moon hanging over the shadow of the fell known as the Old Man of Coniston to the west of the lake. I make a joke about being the Old Woman of Coniston – according to nature and society I am old, as far as having babies is concerned. The man who cannot be named and who is accompanying me on this venture gives me one of those looks when I say this. At eight inches taller and four stone heavier than me, he'd make a much better open-water swimmer than I ever will, but although he loves swimming he doesn't like the cold and is the sort of person who thinks: *If you don't like doing something, why do it?* Why indeed.

Sunday dawns. It's a beautiful day. The lake is shimmering in the morning sun. The water looks inviting and there's no doubt that thinking you want to get in before you remember that you actually don't is the best way to start a swim. We've been told to meet at the Bluebird Café on the north-west shore of the lake for a briefing. It's such a beautiful name and I wistfully think of my alternative weekend, sitting on the terrace with a coffee and a slice of cake, looking out across the water. Instead I join the group congregating outside, where we're talked through the course and the rules. Once this is done we're told to head down to the southern end of the lake where the swim will start at noon. It's quite a long drive to the starting point. I try not to think about the distance.

The rules state that each swimmer has to be escorted by a boat, so there is a lot of faff involved in getting everyone ready for the start. My boat is a canoe which is being paddled by a nice young man called Liam who lives locally. Although it's officially a race I haven't been thinking of it as such until now; my aim has been just to complete it. But while we're waiting, people start stripping down to their swimming costumes and limbering up as if we're at the Olympics. I can't help myself from eyeing up the competition. Most of the swimmers are men but there are a few women, none of whom look particularly fit. I catch myself wondering if I've got any chance in the ladies' category. That would really show Chris and the others.

Finally, the ten-minute whistle goes and the swimmers start to wade out to waist height, their boats in front of them jostling for position. It's a scrum of limbs and paddles in cold water and then the whistle goes again and we're off. The men at the front dive ahead in a thrash of legs and arms. The boats scramble to find their swimmers. If this were a road, there would be rage. I start to swim but within a few seconds of getting going my goggles begin leaking, water seeping in around the edges, so I have to screw up my eyes. I try to push them more tightly onto my face. They leak. I tip them upwards and empty out the water and try again. They still leak. The first few moments in cold water are always disorientating, but the frenzy of swimmers coupled with my leaking goggles unsettle me even more than usual. I don't understand what's happened to them, they were fine last week in the Serpentine. I stop swimming for a moment and look up. Liam is there in his canoe a few feet away, waiting and watching. In the same mortifying second I realise it's just Liam and that everyone else has disappeared. The water is suddenly still. I've not even been swimming for five minutes and I'm last. There's not winning a race, and then there's coming last.

I swim over to the canoe and ask Liam to find me another pair of goggles from my bag. Luckily, I brought a spare but we both know that asking for a new pair of goggles so early on is not a good sign. Leaking goggles are a prophecy that things are not going to go well. I know it. Liam knows it. The other swimmers searing ahead all know it too. My spare goggles don't leak but they are clear, not tinted, and the sun has become so bright that it's now impossible to see. As well as the embarrassment of being so far behind everyone else, I can't even say that I decided to have a leisurely swim and enjoy the majesty of the landscape because everything around me is a blotchy blur. I swim on and try not to think about Chris.

I had agreed with Liam when I was going to take a feed but it begins to feel like such a long time has passed that I'm convinced he must have forgotten. But I don't want to check my watch in case he hasn't and I see that I've still got ages to go until the allotted time. Eventually he gives me the five-minute signal. I start to swim closer to the canoe so that I'm ready the moment he reaches down. But there's more bad news. My brand-new flask, bought at great expense for the occasion and lovingly filled with warm sweet liquid that morning, has cracked. Liam has carefully poured the liquid into a plastic feeding bottle but when he shakes it, it looks like a snow globe. I take a hopeful sip but it's cold and full of shards of glass.

'I don't know what happened,' he says apologetically.

I'm speechless. This is not going well. This is going terribly. I'm last. I'm blind. I'm cold. And now I'm about to starve. I hadn't thought to bring anything else (not even strawberry shoelaces; I've left them on land as my post-swim treat).

'Am I over halfway yet?' I say desperately.

'Definitely,' Liam says.

'How long have I got to go?'

'Half an hour, maybe three-quarters.'

'Am I still last?'

'No.'

'Are you lying?'

'Didn't you see – you overtook some people after your goggles got sorted?'

'No. I can't see a thing,' I say crossly, handing back the snow globe. 'OK, half an hour. Let's do it.'

I start off at a pace, revived not by food but by the news that I've overtaken someone and am no longer last. But the end of the lake doesn't look like it's getting any closer and after what feels like ages I cave in and look at my watch. I've been swimming for another hour. I stop in the water and shout over to Liam: 'We're nowhere near yet. You lied!'

'Yes, we are,' he says. 'See those orange buoys over there, that's the finishing line.'

He points in the distance and I can just make out two orange blobs on the surface of the water.

'No, I can't. I can't see anything,' I shout in the desperate hope that the orange blobs are not what he's pointing to.

'Are you OK?' Liam says. He sounds concerned.

'No,' I snap. 'I might be if I had something to eat.'

I put my head back in the cold water. I know it's not his fault the flask broke and I didn't think to bring anything else, but this is agony to the power of ten. And what am I doing it for anyway? Some vain attempt to prove I've got what it takes to swim the English Channel. But why? It's not like I'm going to be the first person to ever do it, or even the last. I won't be the youngest or the oldest. I'm definitely not going to be the fastest and I may not even be the slowest. Yes, it's big, but it's not going to make any history books or change any lives. It's not like finding the cure for Alzheimer's, is it?

When I finally have about 500 metres or so to go, a rowing boat comes to join Liam to steer me home between them. I find out later that because I couldn't see I had been veering all over the place, and then because the wind had got up even Liam in his small canoe was struggling to keep a straight course beside me. As I wade out of the water, exhausted, I am relieved to have survived the ordeal. But further humiliation is still to come. Back at the Bluebird Café for the race presentation at the end of the afternoon, I suddenly realise that they're not just giving out certificates to the winners; everyone is getting one and our names are being read out loud in the order each of us landed. I feel slightly sick as I wait for my name to be called. I'm not quite last but I am fourth from last, quicker only than a twelve-year-old, an octogenarian and a lady breaststroker. As Chris said, if I ever want to be a Channel swimmer I'm going to have to start taking things seriously. But, after today, do I really want to?

———

The next day, with aching arms, we take Coniston's famous steam gondola out onto the lake to see the route I had swum blindly the day before. It's a beautiful vessel which would be at home in a Canaletto painting and a far superior way to see the lake and her landscape. The gondola drops us off on the eastern shore just below Brantwood, John Ruskin's house. The Victorian polymath bought the property in the latter half of the nineteenth century when he was in poor health, in the hope that bathing in the waters of Coniston would restore him. We climb upwards to explore the house, ending up in the Italianesque turret he had added to the building to provide a magnificent panoramic view of the lake. I look down and imagine Ruskin bathing in the water below and wonder what he would have thought about me swimming from one end to the other. It had been excruciating, but I suppose he is right, there is something about swimming in open water that makes you feel alive. Especially when you get out. It reminds me of my conversation with Susan Greenfield and the word she chose for me. I have no doubt that she would have agreed with Ruskin's famous words: 'There is no wealth but life.'

The Very Reverend

'I wouldn't give up my family for my job.
But I would give up my job for my family.'

Susan Greenfield and Coniston had made me think about life. But the next woman I meet makes me think about death.

Lorna Hood – the Very Reverend – is one of ten honorary chaplains to the queen. She was the first female parish minister in Scotland to hold the esteemed position of Moderator of the General Assembly, one of the most respected roles in the Church. It's an impressive CV, and I have a specific reason for wanting to meet her. I want to talk to Lorna about what she's done for women who have lost babies in pregnancy and childbirth.

She hasn't got long to see me because she's en route from Edinburgh, where she's just done a radio broadcast, to an event in Dundee, and has to catch a train. We arrange to meet near Waverley, the city's central station. I'm thinking the five-star Balmoral Hotel on Princes Street; haggis sandwiches and shortbread with a nip of whisky. But disappointingly she plumps for Costa Coffee, and as

I'm the disciple here, I cordially agree. Not only that, she just wants sparkling water, no food. I like sparkling water, in fact I prefer it to still, but it's not going to help get me across the Channel. I don't seem to be having much luck persuading people to eat with me, and I wonder whether this says something significant about many women's ambivalent relationship with food. Putting that aside for now, I buy her a bottle of water and myself a big slice of chocolate cheesecake. I would never usually do this. Usually, if I was meeting someone who didn't want to eat, I wouldn't eat either. But as the female swimmers at Lake Coniston had demonstrated, fat can be fit, and it's definitely the best way to keep out the cold. So if the women I meet are not going to eat, I figure I better start eating for two. Besides, it's probably the best excuse I'm ever going to have.

I take a mouthful and ask her to tell me the story of how she got involved in pioneering the care of women who had lost their babies during pregnancy and birth. She says it all began when there was a vacancy in the local hospital chaplaincy team. They were looking for someone who would have responsibility for the maternity and special care baby units. As a mother herself and the only member of the presbytery who had any relevant experience, she thought: *I could do this.* She says she spent the first three months going around saying nothing much more than, 'How are you?'

'Then one day,' she says, 'I went into a four-bedded ward and made a silly joke, something like, "Hello, ladies-in-waiting," but when I reached the last woman on the ward, she said to me: "I'm no longer waiting, I lost my baby."'

I put down my fork and stop eating the cheesecake. I know that ward. Four beds, two and two opposite each other. The pervading colours of white and light blue. A window at the end, sealed shut from the cold. The lingering smell of sterility combined with hospital food. Is that the ward she was in, or is it just the one I've been in myself? Because I too know what it's like to be no longer waiting.

'And that's how I got involved,' she continues, her words starting to gather speed, her tone becoming more animated as she describes what happened next. 'It was the best thing I ever did as a hospital chaplain, but it was like opening a can of worms because they just weren't doing anything right. We took the women out of the ward so they weren't with the mothers nursing their babies. We had a special room made. We had handprints, pictures, various things like that done so they didn't leave the hospital with nothing, thinking, "Was I really pregnant?" We got a plot in a cemetery because in the old days the foetus wasn't dealt with in a dignified way, it was just part of the clinical waste. And we also held a memorial service. The first one I gave there were people who had lost a baby forty years before, and afterwards I got so many letters saying, "Thank you. I wasn't allowed to say goodbye." Because it wasn't talked about, people were often told, "Och, you're fine, have another one," but I would do a funeral service for a sixteen-week-old foetus or a baptism if there was a stillbirth. Some of my colleagues totally disagreed with me: they said baptism isn't appropriate because the baby's dead, and I said to them, "I'm not going to have a theological argument with parents who've lost a child. Do you think God is going to be angry with me?"'

She pauses for breath and as she does so I see her glance down at my half-eaten slice of chocolate cheesecake. 'You're tempting me too much,' she says, and picks up the extra fork I brought over just in case and takes some.

I smile the biggest smile and push the plate towards her.

'I don't know God as well as you, but I don't think so,' I say.

———————

Lorna Hood's words have reminded me of my ectopic pregnancy, which was only discovered at three months. It happened after what I believed had been an unsuccessful round of IVF. I'd been bleeding and had taken a test which was negative, so assumed it hadn't worked. But six weeks later I hadn't had another period, which seemed strange, so in secret I took a pregnancy test and to my amazement there was a double line. My immediate thought was that we had conceived naturally – sometimes that happens after IVF – and we were both overjoyed. For a few days we felt like normal people again. But when we went to our doctor for a scan, things deteriorated quickly. He confirmed that I was pregnant, but the pregnancy hormone in my blood was so high that the foetus was much further developed than six weeks, and he couldn't see it in my womb where it was supposed to be. I suddenly found myself being rushed into hospital in what the doctor described quite simply as 'a very dangerous situation'. I was in theatre for over four hours while they looked for the foetus, first in my right fallopian tube, then in my left, until eventually they found it in my stomach. Abdominal ectopics are extremely rare, and later I read about one woman who carried her baby to term although it was born very prematurely. I wished she had been me. But there had been no time to ask any questions. Everything happened so quickly. One minute I was pregnant, the next I was not. Now all I have to show that I was a mother is three small scars across my tummy. I don't even know what happened to the foetus or whether it was a girl or a boy. It haunts me. Was our baby a girl or a boy?

'Lorna,' I say, hoping it's OK to call a Very Reverend by her first name. 'What advice would you give to someone who might not be able to have their own child?'

She puts down the fork and says, 'Look at every avenue possible. Explore every way. Go down every road to find a solution.'

In a way I am surprised by the definitiveness of her response. I had read that she decided to go into the ministry when she was a teenager, so I ask what she would have done if she hadn't been able to conceive herself, whether her vocation would have been enough. She pauses for a long time before answering: 'I don't think so. I lost my parents when I was in my teens and I suppose I wanted someone who was part of me as well. I never considered for a moment that I wouldn't be able to. How I would have coped if that had been the case I honestly don't know. Would it have been enough, or would I have gone down the adoption line? I don't know. I think probably.'

'So can I ask, and please don't answer this if you don't feel comfortable . . .'

'Yes,' she says, as if she's prepared for even the hardest question.

'You're lucky you didn't have that dilemma and you've got two wonderful children *and* your vocation but, how do I phrase this,' I say, fearing the impertinence of my question: 'Are they of equal importance? Of course you don't have to think about it, but if I asked you to think about it, could you choose?'

And without a beat of hesitation she replies: 'I wouldn't give up my family for my job. But I would give up my job for my family.'

I can't help but notice that she calls it her job and not her vocation, and I wonder whether family is the Very Reverend's real vocation, so I ask her what happiness is and she says that it's knowing that she's loved by her husband and her children and being able to give that love back in return.

At the end of our conversation Lorna laughs and says: 'Any word? I could be really rotten and give you the word "eschatological".'

Not rotten at all. Death and the final destiny of the soul and humankind is the perfect word for the Very Reverend to give me to take to sea.

Mother Tallulah

If you had asked me when I was ten years old what I wanted to be when I grew up, I would have said: an actress. My dream was to star on the London stage in *Bugsy Malone*. I would spend hours listening to the soundtrack of the Alan Parker movie. I was always Tallulah, not Blousey. I have found that women are largely divided into Tallulahs and Blouseys, and looking back I wish I were the latter because she ends up with the boy and the happy ending. I tend not to, which is probably why I was Tallulah – strong but slightly sad, as if the glamour of her leading lady life isn't what she truly wanted.

So as a child, having an interesting and impressive job was important to me, but so was having a family. I didn't care much for dolls (I had a Sindy; everyone had a Sindy) but my early maternal instinct came out in a different way – via catalogues. I don't know where I got them from. My mum and dad wouldn't have known where to find a catalogue or what to do with one. But somehow I procured them and I would spend hours picking out the things I was going to buy when I grew up, imagining the life I would lead as an adult. I'd go through each section in turn: women's clothes; men's clothes (I imagined a husband); children's clothes (and toys); homeware; gardening equipment. I remember I'd always choose for myself a pair of those high-heeled fluffy slippers from the nightwear section. Sometimes in black, sometimes in pink. Really, they're the most impractical slipper you could imagine but they seemed to me to be the height of glamour, and as I said, I was Tallulah not Blousey. But there was nothing about this life I was creating from pictures that suggested I wanted to be a 'career woman' as such. What I wanted was a husband, a home and a family, and although I did also want a job, I wasn't sure what it would be. I was cautious about disclosing my theatrical dreams because I knew that you had to be good at singing and dancing to be a musical theatre star and I was never a stage-school kid. I did have tap-dancing lessons for a while but never got beyond a shuffle ball change.

I think back to my conversation with Camila Batmanghelidjh; she had made me wonder whether there are, perhaps, broadly three types of women in the world. In the first category are women who are driven by a vocation, who are either not interested in having children or not particularly disappointed when they don't. Both Camila and the scientist Susan Greenfield seemed to fall into this category. In the second category are women who are purely driven by a maternal instinct, for whom becoming and then being a mother eclipses all other desires. And in the third category there are the women who want both a fulfilling job and motherhood in roughly equal measure. Camila's right, I'm in the third category. The Very Reverend Lorna Hood had seemed to achieve this goal but I was never going to forget her words: 'I wouldn't give up my family for my job. But I would give up my job for my family.' Did this actually put her in category two? And why is that it so often feels as if women have to choose to be in one category or the other, when men don't?

I love my job. I didn't end up acting in the theatre but I did end up running one. It probably sounds more glamorous than it is: my main responsibilities are to ensure that tickets are selling, everyone gets paid, and the (soon to be fully tiled) loos are not blocked in the morning. But it is a great job and throughout my twenties I worked very hard for it. The question that keeps coming back to me, however, is: is it enough on its own? Am I doing what Camila had levelled at me, living my life authentically, or just making do with what I've got? Do I need to do what Lorna said and go down every avenue possible to become a mother if I want to be truly happy?

I think back to my ten-year-old self with her catalogues, dreaming of being Tallulah. I wonder what I would have chosen if some fairy godmother had granted me one wish with the words: 'Jessica, you can either grow up and be an actress as feted and successful as Marilyn Monroe, or I'll guarantee you a house, a husband, four children (two girls and two boys) and everything you've put a cross next to in that catalogue of yours. But, Jessica, there's one condition: you can only have one of them. Which one will you choose?'

I look at my fairy godmother. She's dressed in pink sparkly net. She looks like Glinda, the Good Witch of the

North in *The Wizard of Oz*. And I say to her: 'But what if I can't choose, fairy godmother? What happens to girls who want to be both? What happens to girls who want to be Mother Tallulah?'

And I guess my deepest fear is that she looks at me and says: 'Jessica, I'm afraid it's been decided. *You* cannot be both.'

The Ballerina

'I am conscious that I'm not hitched to anyone else's wagon.'

We meet at the Delaunay, the glamorous pseudo-nineteenth-century Viennese coffee house on the corner of London's Aldwych. I order *Sachertorte* – in honour of Vienna – and she orders a lemon meringue tart.

'So the dancer eats cake!' I exclaim.

'Don't start!' she says, her tone half harsh, half humorous.

I wince with embarrassment. I guess I could lie and say that the last woman I'd met hadn't wanted to eat at all and the one before that had only eaten a teaspoonful, and that my delight was somehow linked to this. But that wouldn't be the truth: we both immediately recognise how cringingly crass my comment is. Thankfully, she seems to forgive me when I say how mortified I am and proceeds to tell me an anecdote about the stage doorkeeper at the Royal Opera House who would often have a stash of chocolates that had been sent in as gifts for dancers and singers and would always say something similar whenever she came by and took one: 'He'd say, "Ooh, you're having a chocolate."' She mimics the conversation using the same tone for him as I have just used when commenting on her ordering a cake. 'And then I'd say: "It's fine for you to say that to me, but you do realise if you say that to somebody with a sensitive attitude you could just have triggered an episode of a serious eating disorder."'

I can imagine Deborah Bull, former principal of the Royal Ballet, ticking off the stage doorkeeper brusquely like this. She is definitely a woman who knows how to speak her mind. Towards the end of her ballet career she was invited to the Oxford Union to oppose the motion 'This House believes that the National Lottery gives too much support to the elitist arts'. You have to admire anyone who is prepared to stand up and defend the charitable merits of ballet and opera over more obviously worthy causes, but by all accounts her appearance was a triumph. For her, it marked the beginning of a realisation that she could do something beyond ballet and, following her retirement from dancing, she has become a high-profile cultural commentator and campaigner. It is impossible not to be impressed by the breadth of her achievements, but the one thing she doesn't have on her CV is motherhood.

I first heard Deborah Bull talk about this on my all-time favourite Radio 4 programme, *Desert Island Discs*. The thing which had most intrigued me was that when she was asked about not having children she'd said, in that piercing way I have experienced myself, that she may not be a mother, but that didn't mean she didn't understand motherhood, because although she doesn't have a 'downwards' family she does have an 'upwards' one. Unfortunately she wasn't asked to elaborate on what she meant, because I really wanted to hear more.

Our tea (and calories) arrives: fresh-leafed and served in a beautiful silver pot which comes with a technically challenging tea-strainer that takes quite a bit of working out. Hopeless at doing two things at the same time, I endeavour to get Deborah talking as I try to master it.

'So, did motherhood ever figure for you?' I ask.

'No, it didn't,' she says quickly. 'I can honestly say, at no point. I was married briefly and it sort of occurred to me that it would be an option, but really that's as far as it went. It's never been something I've agonised about or deeply analysed, it's just always seemed clear that it's not held any attraction.'

So that's that then. Here's another woman, like Susan Greenfield, who genuinely doesn't seem that bothered that she didn't become a mother. Deborah Bull is in category one. We talk on, discussing the difficulties of being a dancer and having to give up your vocation at a relatively young age, and whether it's possible to have two vocations in one life. We talk about whether Deborah should go into politics (she should go into politics) and how hard it is, because you need to have the hide of a rhinoceros (she definitely doesn't have the hide of a rhinoceros). We talk about her desire to reach a Buddhist state of calm without practising Buddhism. 'Wish me luck with that,' she laughs. And then, finally, I ask her the question I most want to know the answer to: what had she meant by her 'upwards' family?

'For me a deep realisation came when my mother died,' she says. 'It was the most profoundly life-changing moment. For most of my life I'd been used to a world where the Swan Queen died every night and got up again. My mother's death was my first real understanding of mortality and my remaining upward family became much more important to me as a consequence. I actually moved house so I could be nearer to my dad. And I became very concerned with getting people together. I remember once trying to organise a party for his birthday and being very pernickety about the details. Everything had to be perfect. At one point I said to my sisters, "Look, I'm really sorry, but you have to understand this is the only family I've got." And they said, "Yes, Deb, we've clocked that."'

I smile, understanding all too well the desire to make things perfect that are not, but I'm also fascinated by what she says about family.

She takes a sip of tea and then continues. 'So when I'm asked about not having children, I talk about my upwards family because I think there's a sort of feeling sometimes that, "Oh, you wouldn't understand, you're outside the club," and I think: "No, I do. I do understand. I have been one half of the parent–child relationship. I haven't been the other half. But I have been one half of it. So don't say I don't understand, because I sort of do . . ."'

Again Deborah's words remind me of my conversation with Susan Greenfield. I had asked Susan what she felt her greatest achievements were and she'd said that, undoubtedly, the biggest was introducing her mum to the Queen. What struck me about this was that before speaking to her I had read an interview that she and her mother, Doris, had done for a newspaper in which Doris said her proudest moment as Susan's mother had been meeting the Queen. There was such poignancy in this. Susan, like Deborah, had done an excellent job of convincing me that being childless had not been a particular sadness or disappointment for her, yet it was still an expression of the love between mother and daughter that she chose as her greatest achievement. And now Deborah describes her mother's death as her most profoundly life-changing moment. What seems important here is that even if a woman is not a parent she still understands the nature of that love – the love *of* a parent, the love *for* a parent. So why is it that society doesn't seem to want to accept that a childless woman can love like a mother? Emboldened by her honesty, I ask whether she's ever had any regrets about not having her own 'downwards family', which would of course have legitimised the love of her upwards one.

'No,' she says firmly, 'but there is something that has recently struck me about the trajectory of life.'

'Yes?' I say, eager for insight.

'It's a long great big mountain that you climb up and then you get to a point when you realise it's just as steep on the other side and you're going to go down really, really quickly towards the end. It seems to me that there's a trick to avoid that, which is to have a child and hitch your wagon to someone else who is on the way up. Live it all again in the slipstream. And some people do that really brilliantly and the kids are happy to have them along, and some kids are like: "Bugger off, it's not your wagon . . ."'

We both laugh.

'So no regrets,' she says, 'but I am conscious that I'm not hitched to anyone else's wagon.'

A journalist once wrote that Deborah Bull has the eloquence of a ballerina, and she does. I could talk to her beyond tea and into supper but I'm conscious that she has another meeting to go to and we need to wrap up. So I ask her my last question.

'Oh gosh, one word . . . I'm not sure any of my favourite words are useful here,' she says. 'I love the word "integrity" and the word "rigour" . . .' She pauses for a moment to think and then says, 'I know. I'll give you the word "ruth". As in the opposite of "ruthless".'

———————

As I walk home, I think about Deborah's word and wonder why it is used so little in comparison to its antonym. When I get in I decide to look it up in the dictionary. The entry reads: '"ruth", pronounced "rooth", meaning "compassion" or "pity".' Maybe she's telling me that I need to have compassion for myself. Does she mean in my pursuit of motherhood? Or in my quest to swim the Channel to make up for not being a mother? I hope she's not giving me her pity. And as I sit thinking this through I am struck by the fact that this is the second biblical word I've been given. It derives from the story of Ruth and Naomi in the Old Testament:

when Naomi loses her two sons she tries to persuade her daughters-in-law, Orpah and Ruth, to leave her and go back to their own families. But Ruth refuses with the words: 'Entreat me not to leave thee, or to return from following after thee; for whither thou goest, I will go, and where thou lodgest, I will lodge. Thy people shall be my people, and thy God my God.'

It is Ruth's profound act of loyalty to the older woman that defines the meaning of the word. And I wonder if I am Naomi and this journey I'm on is about finding my Ruth, who will let me hitch my wagon in the slipstream of her life.

Molly

My Ruth is called Molly. She can swim like a fish. She's clever and kind and funny like her dad, and determined and spirited and sometimes even funnier than her dad, like her mum. My Ruth is called Molly and she lived with us for nine weeks inside my womb. Until she died.

A few months after our ectopic pregnancy, we went for another round of IVF. We had two frozen embryos left over from our last treatment. This time things went the way they should, at least to begin with. On 'official test day' I took a pregnancy test and it was positive. I remember ringing the clinic, like you're told to, and saying the words but not really believing they could actually be true. They congratulated me warmly. I didn't believe their congratulations either. But over the next few days, I took test after test to reassure myself and each time there they were: the double lines of happiness.

At our first six-week scan there were signs that things weren't quite right. As I lay on the hospital trolley with the scanning probe inside me, I watched as the nurse stared at the screen doing something that made a repetitive clicking sound. After what felt like forever she turned to us and said there was good news and bad. The good news was that she could see a strong heartbeat, but the bad news was the foetus was around half the size it should be at this stage in gestation. The clicking sound had been her measuring it. She turned the screen towards us to show us the tiny fluttering spot, fighting for its life.

For years we had dreamed of having a little girl called Molly. It's the only name we've ever both agreed on. So we named her Mini-Molly and with all the hope in our hearts willed for her to keep growing. At our second scan she had doubled in size – Mini-Molly was now nine millimetres and we left the clinic with one of those grainy black-and-white photos of a jellybean-shaped dot that was our little girl. But still things weren't quite right; I had been spotting on and off, which is never a good sign.

At our next scan, although she was still there, Mini-Molly's heartbeat had stopped. For over a week I willed that the nurse had made a mistake and the miscarriage she predicted would never come. But it did – at a West End theatre during a Saturday matinee. I'll never forget standing in the queue for the toilets at the interval, closing the cubicle door, and the massive rush of blood.

Since my conversation with Deborah Bull, I've been thinking a lot about why it's so important to some humans to have their own children. This wasn't our first miscarriage; we'd had two before from our first and second rounds of IVF, although they had happened very early on and were technically known as 'biochemical pregnancies', where the embryo implants in the uterus momentarily but doesn't take hold. Our third round of IVF was negative, the fourth resulted in our ectopic, and this miscarriage happened after our fifth. So why did we keep going back for more when something clearly wasn't working? It was partly because every doctor we saw was convinced that the fact I could get pregnant was a good sign and that if we kept on trying it would eventually happen. And partly it was because of a determination not to accept defeat. Yet we could have started to think about alternative routes to parenthood earlier – adoption, fostering, or egg or embryo donation. We could have looked for Ruth a long time ago. But we didn't; we wanted to create our own biological child – our Mini-Molly.

Why do humans have this atavistic desire? It's not like the planet needs any more people, and there are so many children that desperately need a loving home. So why do people feel the need to hitch their wagon to children of their own? Someone said to me once, it's 'genetic imperialism' – an urge to propagate the world with ourselves. But I think it's often a far less confident gesture than that. I think a massive part of wanting your own genetically related child is so you can live your own life again, especially your childhood. For me, having children is less about demonstrating our physiological power and more about healing our psychological pain. And when you can't have children, or you lose the ones that might have been, your deepest fear is that you may never get a chance to live the life you've always wanted for yourself. I needed Mini-Molly in the world far more than she ever needed me.

A Few Words on Jellyfish

If there's one thing that is starting to worry me about the Channel more than the cold, it's the jellyfish. I'd never given these gelatinous creatures much thought in the past apart from after one of our early unsuccessful rounds of IVF, when me and the man whose name starts with a consonant took a road trip along Highway 1 from Los Angeles to San Francisco. Sometimes unsuccessful rounds of IVF can have unintended positives, although beware, compensatory holidays like this also increase the credit card debt. It wasn't the trip where I wrote my bucket list. That was later. That was Gambia. (We were rapidly running out of money by then and you can get really cheap package deals there – it's like the Costa del Sol of Africa.)

But back to the jellyfish. En route north we stopped off at Monterey and visited the famous aquarium there, and they had these beautiful bright blue illuminated tanks with translucent coral-coloured jellyfish wafting across them. And the man whose name does not start with a vowel stood filming them as their bodies contracted rhythmically in and out. When we got back to England he put a soundtrack to the footage and for months, every night when I got home from work, he'd have those jellyfish on the telly with their jellyfish music. He'd go on and on about how beautiful they were and I would harrumph because admiring the jellyfish didn't pay off the credit card debt. Of course I had no idea then that they'd become my future nemesis.

There are two ways that animals can harm humans chemically. The first is by poison and the second by venom. Poisonous animals can be passive, but if you eat or touch them you're going to get sick. Venomous creatures are more actively aggressive. They bite, stab or sting you. In the case of jellyfish they shoot little hypodermic needles from their tentacles into your skin. Once their venom is inside you, it hurts. Sometimes it hurts a lot. Sometimes it can kill you.

The number of jellyfish off the coast of the UK is growing, as a result of global warming. This means that the Channel is probably warmer than when Matthew Webb and Gertrude Ederle swam it, but it also means that I'm more likely to encounter a smack. A smack is the collective noun for jellyfish – like a shoal of fish or a pod of dolphins. I know which collective noun I'd rather meet.

Although there are hundreds of different jellyfish around the world, there are only six commonly found off the UK coast: the moon, the compass, the lion's mane, the barrel, the blue and the mauve stinger. None of them will kill you, but who wants to even say hello? It's said that Channel swimmers are most likely to encounter jellyfish in the separation zone, the strip of sea that divides the north and south shipping lanes. Maybe they congregate there to chat, to avoid the tankers and ferries. About five hundred vessels plough up and down the English Channel each day. It's another hazard of the swim – but a boat, whilst dangerous, is much easier to avoid than a smack in the face.

For every jellyfish tale you hear, there's also a remedy: vinegar, 'meat tenderiser' (what is meat tenderiser?) and plain old pee. I don't relish the thought of any of them and am just praying that no jellyfish are planning on heading my way. I guess I should just be thankful for the fact that the Channel's too cold for sharks. There are other open-water swims around the world where the water may be warmer but you have to swim in a cage if you don't want to get eaten. Some crazy open-water swimmers even forgo the cage. So there may be jellyfish in the Channel but the fact that there aren't any sharks has got to be a bonus. And, besides, as open-water swimmers are wont to say: 'The sea is our playground and their home,' which roughly translates as: 'They've got every right to be there and we haven't.'

I've not yet been able to think of the sea as my playground, but I'm working on it. I really am.

Team Toe Dip

We've called ourselves 'Team Toe Dip'. It was almost 'Just Add Water' and, when the day comes, on the drive down to Dover, I have a crisis about the name.

'Do you think we chose the right one?' I ask.

'Too late now,' Dom says, 'we're on our way.'

It is. We are.

———

I had hastily assembled a team of three people for the relay: me; my best friend's brother-in-law, Steve; and his mate, Dom. It was all a bit ad hoc. Over a drink I had mentioned that I was hoping to swim the Channel next year. Steve was interested and impressed because he's done a bit of open-water swimming himself, and then when the slot came up I approached him and he approached Dom, who I'd never met before, and soon we were a threesome. I knew it was quite a small number of people for a relay but I figured it would be a good test, and after Coniston I hoped that a few hour-long legs in the sea punctuated by food and rest on the boat was doable, even for me.

At four on the Friday afternoon of our tidal week I got the call from our pilot telling us to be in Dover harbour the following morning at seven. This time I wasn't going to make the same mistake as at Coniston, and I'd prepared a list of things to bring for every eventuality, especially on the food front. It's ironic, but it felt a bit like I was an expectant mother with a hospital bag checklist. As soon as word came that water was about to break, I got out my list and ran through it.

1. Cool box
2. Flask – non-breakable
3. Ham & cheese baguette
4. Peanut butter & jam baguette
5. Chicken pot noodles
6. Banana bread
7. Trail mix
8. White chocolate
9. Strawberry shoelaces
10. Energy gels
11. Maxim carbohydrate and fruit squash
12. Water
13. Green tea
14. Coffee (one-cup filters)
15. Swimming bag
16. Swimming costumes – several
17. Goggles (clear and tinted)
18. Hat

19. Ear plugs
20. Towel
21. Dryrobe
22. Sleeping bag
23. Crocs
24. Black leggings
25. Grey jumper
26. Grey jacket
27. Socks
28. Hat
29. Waterproofs
30. Passport
31. Insurance details
32. Suncream
33. Sunglasses

Everything was ready. I just had to make the banana bread and buy a fresh baguette from the corner shop on my way home from work. I'd come up with the banana bread idea a few weeks ago but I have to admit the idea of baking was losing ground rapidly. All I really wanted to do was go home and sleep because I was going to have to be up at four. But I wanted the day to be perfect – just like Deborah Bull wanted for her dad's birthday – and I had this picture of myself eating banana bread on the deck of the boat, fresh from the second leg of my swim (after the first leg I'd already decided I was going to have the peanut butter and jam baguette). So as soon as I got home I forced myself into the kitchen and started mashing bananas.

———————

And now we're in the car, heading east out of London. The dawning day looks like it's going to be beautiful, and just to make things even more perfect, my best friend, Tara – Steve's sister-in-law – is with us too. This is serendipity because she now lives in Australia and there was only one day on her whirlwind trip to the UK when she was going to be able to come with us. We didn't know exactly which day we'd be going because it depends on the weather and the other swimmers in your tidal week (each pilot has four swimming slots per tide and as we were a cancellation we were the last). But the stars of the sea have aligned and Tara is able to join us. Everyone is delighted as you couldn't get a better crew member. She's a firefighter, a trained physiotherapist and a surfboat rower, which means that she's got great sea legs, knows how to relieve a shoulder injury and can give mouth-to-mouth if required.

We arrive at the harbour in good time, park the car, get out our things and head down to the jetty where our boat and pilot are waiting. There's an expression on his face that I can't decipher at first, but I sense something's not quite right, and when we get on board he tells us that the forecast isn't looking favourable later and the sea may be too rough to swim. We're all disappointed. There is only one more day left in this week's tide and there's no guarantee the weather will be any better tomorrow. We sit out on the deck discussing the situation. I make everyone a coffee using my one-cup filters. No one can quite believe I've gone to the effort of bringing fresh coffee but it was another of my attempts to make things perfect. I get out the banana bread and offer everyone a slice. Time slows down for a while as we sit around with no clear idea of what to do next. Then suddenly our pilot, who has been on and off the boat conversing with harbour colleagues, gets back on board and says that it looks like the weather has settled a bit and some of the other boats have decided to go.

I look at the boys. The boys look at me. Then a group of people jump onto the boat that is moored alongside ours and start the engine. A woman in the group takes off her jacket and poses for a photograph in her swimming costume with an American flag. The boat starts to move out of the harbour. They've clearly decided to go and she looks like a soloist. I've been told relayers can generally take a bit more risk with the weather because it's a group effort.

'Let's do it,' I say. 'Let's do this Channel thing.'

The boys agree.

No one swims out of the harbour itself. Your support boat takes you along the coastline to one of two starting points: either Shakespeare Beach or Samphire Hoe. About one hundred metres from land, the boat stops and then the swimmer (or in the case of a relay, the first swimmer) jumps out, swims to shore, clears the water and stands on the beach until a claxon sounds, signalling the start. With relays your strongest swimmer goes first. In our case that's Dom. He'll be followed by Steve, and then me. The aim is to swim in this order in succession all the way to France.

It's quite emotional seeing Dom standing on the beach

waiting for the claxon. I feel a rush of nervous anticipation, which is less about the swim ahead of us and more about the thought that next year it could be me standing on the shore, facing a solo. But that's next year. Today the sun is out, the sky is blue and the sea seems fairly calm to me. Just after Dom starts swimming a seal appears to wish us luck. It's going to be a perfect day.

———

The first time I'm sick is after my initial leg in the water. The swim itself had been fine. I'd jumped off the back of the boat and as per the official rules swum behind Steve until I'd overtaken him and then kept on going for an hour, until I was called in. Tara was doing a great job of helping everyone. It was difficult getting dressed on a rocking boat, shivering from the cold, and she would pass us our towels and clothes and then make us a hot drink. She had poured me a cup of tea and asked what I wanted to eat. That was the point at which I realised that I wasn't hungry; I was going to be sick.

The sea is definitely getting rougher the further out we get, but the added problem is that a little boat going very slowly to keep pace with a swimmer gets buffeted about whatever the weather. I'd heard about people getting sick on the support boat – Andy had first mentioned it in Formentera – but had I listened? No. I'd never been seasick before in my life so I naively assumed I'd be fine. Just go back to that long list of things I brought with me and you'll note that there is nothing on it that remotely resembles seasickness tablets. Absobloodylutely nothing.

As I lean over the side of the boat, banana bread spatters the wind like abstract art. Tara scrapes my hair back to keep it out of the way of the Jackson Pollock. I sit back.

'I don't think I'll be eating that banana bread again in a hurry.'

'That's all right,' Tara says. 'I'll finish it – it's delicious. And who knew that when I was holding your head over that toilet when we were sixteen, it was all in training for today!'

I laugh. Tara and I went through a lot together when we were growing up. We shared our first car – a cream Mini – which I crashed the day after we got it (she took it well); we went island-hopping together in Greece after our A levels (the only way to come of age is with ouzo); and we spent endless teenage nights talking, laughing, crying, drinking, smoking and, yes, occasionally being sick.

The two-hour gap between my first and second swims passes more quickly than it feels it should. After I've got changed, tried to have something to eat and drink, been sick, laid on the deck of the boat recovering and been sick again, it is nearly time to get back in. I am marginally encouraged when Steve says he's heard that some people are less nauseous in the water than out of it, but at the same time getting back in is not a thought I'm relishing on any level. When the time finally comes, I jump off the back again and start swimming. The sea is much rougher than it was on my first leg but I carry on, trying my best to keep up with the boat. I see what I'm sure is the shadow of a jellyfish but thankfully, the waves take it off in another direction and it doesn't come too close.

After me, Dom is in again and we are now into our seventh hour, but the conditions have worsened and, according to our pilot, our pace has slowed down considerably. It's raining, seawater is spilling over the side of the boat, and Dom is swimming, but he's mainly going up and down on the waves and not forward. The boat is hardly moving at all. Actually, that's not true; it's rocking all over the place, it's just not moving forward.

When I've got changed, Tara asks me what I want to eat but I don't feel like anything. She urges me to have something to keep my energy levels up and eventually, I agree to give the chicken noodles a go. She makes them up and brings them over. I take one mouthful, then throw up over the boat. This is now officially not the perfect day I was imagining. It's – what's that word again – AGONY! The pilot comes out of the captain's cabin to ask what we want to do; apparently the boat with the American has turned back. I know I don't want to give up, but at the same time I'm hating every second. He tells us the conditions are just going to get worse and we're going so slowly it could take well over twenty hours to get there. Both Steve and I feel it wouldn't be right to make the decision without Dom, so we agree to wait until he finishes his latest leg to see what he thinks. Our pilot goes back into the cabin. I lay down on the deck of the boat, feeling wretched. A few minutes later another massive wave crashes over us and the pilot rushes out.

'That's it,' he shouts. 'I'm calling the swim. It's getting too dangerous.'

Quickly and without discussion, he goes over to the side of the boat and waves his hands to get Dom's attention. Dom looks up. The pilot starts beckoning him in furiously. Dom swims to the back of the boat and climbs up the steps. He doesn't protest. We all know there's nothing we can do. What the pilot says goes. Our Channel relay attempt, six and a half hours in, is over.

Slowly, the boat turns round, picks up speed and starts heading back to Dover. I sit huddled in the hull, feeling angry and defeated. The sea was rough, but did our pilot call the swim too early? Why weren't we given the opportunity to discuss it more as a team? I start to concoct conspiracy theories that after the pilot had seen me swimming he thought we were going to take too long and he wanted to get back so he could have a good night's sleep. Maybe the weather forecast is looking better tomorrow and he has some other swimmers lined up. There's no second chance once a Channel attempt has been officially registered, which usually takes place within an hour of setting off from Dover. Six and half hours is a bona fide attempt and we are also going to have to pay the full fee for the boat, which isn't cheap.

Later that evening we learn that four of the five boats that made the decision to go at the same time as us didn't get across. I phone Boris and Nick from the Serpentine, who are incredulous that any boats set out at all and tell me we shouldn't have gone. I should probably have consulted them before we went but they still intimidate me, and I'd been all English about it, not wanting to bother them.

None of this changes the fact that our relay ended before we'd even really got started. I'd swum for a total of two hours, which is even less than I'd swum in Lake Coniston. Two hours doesn't even touch the sides of a solo attempt, but it had still been a pretty gruesome introduction. I suppose the only good thing is that it's just as well we called ourselves Team Toe Dip – we hardly even got wet.

Frankenstein Dreaming

In the aftermath of our relay, I have a shocking revelation: swimming the Channel is the same as going through fertility treatment. However hard you try, in the end, whether you're successful or not isn't in your control. There are forces at work that are beyond you, and however good a swimmer you are, however hard you train, however much you want it, you may not make it across. Failure is as much a possibility as success; in fact, it's probably more of a possibility than success. Swimming the English Channel is just like IVF.

In 1978, newspaper articles around the world proclaimed that Mary Shelley's monster had arrived – the Frankenstein myth had become a reality. In fact, she was a baby girl called Louise Brown, who was born at Oldham General Hospital, near Manchester. Her mother and father, Lesley and John, had been trying to conceive for many years and on 25 July 1978 they became the world's first IVF parents. But little Louise really had four parents. Her very own

Frankensteins were two doctors: scientist Robert Edwards and gynaecologist Patrick Steptoe.

Following her birth, Louise became the most famous baby in the world overnight. Lesley and John were mobbed by journalists and had to go into hiding. It's said that they were overwhelmed by the public interest and hadn't fully realised that Louise was going to be the first baby born as a result of reproduction without sex. Apart from Jesus, of course – and there were many who believed that baby Louise must be either superhuman or subhuman and accused her creators of playing God.

But Louise's birth wasn't really a modern miracle, as many have since described it. Edwards and Steptoe had been working tirelessly for years, largely in secret, to make it happen. Initially, their work was so controversial they had to use their own sperm in their experiments. They also enlisted the help of childless couples who volunteered to take part in trials in the hope that these two men could somehow make their dream of a family come true. Lesley and John were among them, but in all the excitement around Louise's birth the others who paved the way for her and for whom it didn't work have been long forgotten. Most of them would be in their late seventies and eighties by now. I wonder whether they found parenthood or whether they were forever science's rejects: the mice that didn't make it.

Louise's birth was a major milestone in medical history. Since then over five million IVF babies have been born around the world. They are no longer making headlines and assisted conception has become so ubiquitous that it's now seen by many as the modern way of making babies. When Louise was growing up there was no question that she was 'different', but nowadays children conceived in Petri dishes (they were never made in test tubes) are everywhere. Many of them may not even know that they started life in a laboratory.

Robert Edwards, shunned by the world at first, was awarded the Nobel Prize for medicine in 2010, just a few years before he died. Patrick Steptoe never received that accolade; he'd died twenty years earlier, when the science was still developing and people were highly suspicious of what it meant. Nowadays there's no question that these two men are responsible for one of the most important scientific and societal developments of our times, along with the world's first embryologist, Jean Purdy – so often forgotten, probably because she was a woman – who assisted Edwards and Steptoe in their pioneering work. Together these three did what Captain Matthew Webb had done when he crossed the English Channel unaided in 1875 – they achieved what seemed impossible.

The phenomenal success and growth of IVF means you'd be forgiven for thinking that it's a guaranteed cure for infertility. And it is incredible – but it doesn't work every time, for everyone. Roughly two-thirds of all treatment cycles fail – statistics that haven't changed much since Louise Brown was born. Whilst this is shocking, it's not surprising, because IVF just helps to make sure that everything is in the right place at the right time; it can't cheat nature completely. Even young, fully fertile couples don't get pregnant every month they try to conceive. So while the world may be full of IVF babies, it's also full of people who have given it a shot and been disappointed. Sometimes they try again and it works. Sometimes they try eleven times and it doesn't.

———

The powerlessness you feel when you realise that no amount of money and medicine will give you a baby is hard to live with. And like the women in the early days of the experiments in Oldham, those of us who for whom fertility treatment fails today are often forgotten about. As were the women who had been through miscarriage and stillbirth on the wards that the Very Reverend Lorna Hood had visited. But maybe we're all still mothers, even when society says that we're not – it's just that our motherhood stories ended in loss.

Now it seems I have chosen to do something else which, just like IVF, I'm statistically more likely to fail at than succeed. What our relay taught me was not whether I wanted to or could do a solo. It taught me that, just like IVF, nature is ultimately in control of this challenge, not me. In the end I can't control my body, and I can't control the sea.

The Polar Explorer

'You have to look at the blessings in life.'

Today the sun is shining on Waterloo Bridge as I make my way to the train station. But when I get there I'm mortified to find that my station sandwich stalwart has made a dreadful decision.

'You've halved the size of it,' I say to the man on the other side of the counter, pointing at the sausage baguette.

He tells me it's company orders.

'But why? It was a perfect size before.' My tone is indignant as my mind starts to frantically run through all the other food options on the station. There are only seven minutes until my train departs.

The man behind the counter can obviously read the panic in my face so suggests I take two and he'll give me a 20 per cent discount. I rally in an instant. There's only one thing better than a sausage sandwich on a train in the morning and that's two sausage sandwiches.

By the time I reach Exeter it's nearly time for lunch and I'm almost hungry again. I make my way along the high street to the appointed restaurant and explain to the manager who greets me at the door that I'm meeting someone I've never met before and I'm not sure whether they've arrived yet.

'Ooh', he says, intrigued. 'Is it a blind date?'

'Kind of', I say.

'Ooh', he says again.

'Can we have a quiet table?'

'Of course!' he says unctuously. 'Upstairs will be best. Why don't you go and get settled and I'll send him up as soon as he arrives.'

'Her', I correct him.

'Oh, I'm sorry', he says, looking embarrassed at his assumption.

'That's OK', I smile. 'And just to confuse you even further, she's going to be with her daughter.'

This time he just nods silently so as not to make another mistake.

When I wrote to the polar explorer Ann Daniels, I'd mentioned my Channel challenge but had added in parentheses, 'I realise it in no way compares to the extraordinary expeditions you've been on.' She wrote back the same day and said: 'I'm impressed with anyone who takes on the sea', and, to my delight, agreed to meet me in Exeter, which is the nearest city to the Devon village where she lives. Her words made my day but I did wonder whether she was just being nice – there's Channel cold and there's Arctic cold, and surely they're poles apart.

I want to talk to Ann about keeping warm, but I am also fascinated by her journey to motherhood. In 1994, Ann gave birth to IVF triplets. She'd been told that there was a less than

15 per cent chance that one of the three embryos transferred to her womb would take hold. But all of them did. Then, just eighteen months after they were born, she left them to go to the North Pole, where she became part of the first all-female relay expedition to reach ninety degrees north. She was on the first leg of the relay and so didn't have the chance to get to the pole herself, but she came back a few years later and triumphed as part of the first all-female team to go the whole way together. And then in 2007 she went back again in an attempt, which ultimately failed, to become the first woman to do it solo. She has consistently made media headlines as the mum of triplets turned polar explorer (and following the birth of Sarah, her youngest, who is joining us for lunch, she is now a mum of four). But oftentimes there has been an undercurrent of media criticism that a mother would choose to leave her children for months at a time for a personal pursuit, especially after she struggled so hard to have them. I want to know why she felt that she needed to do it. I want to know whether it is because motherhood is sometimes not enough.

When she arrives, the first thing that strikes me about Ann is that she's one of those people who radiates fitness and seems much younger than her fifty years. With such a petite frame and so little fat on her my first question has to be: how does she cope with the cold? She tells me you just have to put it in a box. Maybe that's my problem, I've not been carrying a box – but I don't say this. Instead I ask whether she also puts on weight before each expedition. She tells me that in the lead-up she treats it like a job, putting on weight and doing as much training as she can.

'I prefer the eating to the training,' I confess.

'But you've got to do everything to make this feat you're attempting a success,' she says. 'Because if you fail – and with things like the Channel and the North Pole there's more chance of failing than succeeding – then at least you'll know that you've done all you could.'

This is good advice. There are people who wing it through life – it's not a bad way to be and I've been guilty of a bit of flying myself from time to time – but they're not the sort of people who swim the Channel or get to the North Pole. It may help to carry a box, but you also need to make sure that you've put plenty in it before you set out.

At this point a waitress comes over. Ann's ten-year-old daughter, Sarah, orders a main of chicken skewers with couscous and then goes back to her iPad, which has kept her quietly distracted all the time we've been talking. Ann opts for a starter portion of crab cakes as her main (yes, a starter portion – I told you she was trim). Given my breakfast bonus earlier, I decide to do the same.

'So, can I ask, what do you do if you've done everything you can and then fail through no fault of your own? How do you cope with that?' I tell her my recent Channel relay story, but am also aware there's the subtext of my IVF failure. Ann tells me that she had a similar situation on her solo. She spent two years raising the sponsorship money, then a year of training, but when she finally got there, the Russians swooped in, removed everyone's permit and pulled her off the ice after twenty-one days and 175 miles.

'That must have been terrible,' I acknowledge.

'I sat in the helicopter and I was devastated. It felt like three years of my life had been taken away from me and there was nothing I could do about it. But then I thought, hang on a minute, Ann, you've had the adventure of a lifetime. You've managed to spend twenty-one days on the ice on your own and have had five encounters with polar bears. There are so many people who would never get to do any of this. You have to look at the blessings in life.'

I notice as she says this she touches a chain around her neck, which I see for the first time has a silver polar bear hanging from it.

Our lunch arrives and we chat on. One of the things that strikes me most about Ann as I learn more about her life is that she has endured a lot of sadness and disappointment. A difficult childhood; a long struggle to have children (due to what she describes as having only one mangled tube and half an ovary); a broken marriage (to the father of her triplets – Sarah is the daughter from her second husband); and most recently one of the triplets has been very ill. Her life has not been an easy one in any way, and yet she seems to be someone who appreciates what it's given her in spite of the sadness. And even when her dream of becoming the first woman to reach the pole solo didn't materialise, she focused on the fact that she'd had the opportunity to get there at all and experience one of the most magnificent places on earth.

The waitress comes over to clear our plates and ask if we want puddings or coffee. Sarah, on my encouragement, chooses chocolate fudge cake (way to go, Sarah). Ann and

I are more abstemious and order coffees: a flat white for her, a cappuccino for me. The waitress asks whether I want chocolate on the top (of course I want chocolate on the top). I wonder what to ask Ann next. I'm conscious that we've hardly talked about motherhood and I haven't broached the question I came to ask. Does it make you happy – is it enough? But her experiences as a polar explorer are so fascinating, I want to know more. Could it be that the answer is in the conversation?

'So talk to me about polar bears,' I say instead.

Ann smiles: 'Well, I'd never seen any on my previous expeditions and I saw five on my solo, although mainly from a distance. But this one,' she touches the silver polar bear round her neck again, 'this one is *my* bear.' She then recounts an extraordinary story of how she was sitting half dressed in her tent one morning having breakfast when a dark shadow fell across it. At first she told herself that it was nothing, that she was imagining things. But when she looked out she saw a polar bear standing five feet away on its hind legs, facing her. Ann points to the table beside ours to indicate just how near it was. She was carrying a gun for such eventualities but felt as terrified for the bear's life as she did for her own. The last thing she wanted to do was kill it. So, shaking, she scrambled for her gun, and shot the ice just to the side of it. The polar bear looked down, then looked at Ann, but didn't move. Then, after a few seconds, it dropped onto all fours, which Ann says she knew was when a polar bear was at its most dangerous. She shot at it again, this time just above its head, and it moved away. But all day it followed her at distance, watching. The next day it appeared again, then again the day after, each time following and watching. And then, on the third day, it disappeared.

Later, when she was lifted off the ice and got back to base camp, she described what had happened. It transpired that one of the other expedition teams who was not far in front of her had had an encounter with a polar bear on the same three days. On the third day, when one of the men on the team had gone off behind a ridge with a shovel to do what men do behind ridges with shovels, the polar bear had come right up to him. In defence he had hit the bear round the head with said shovel and it had run off. After that none of them saw it again. Ann laughs: 'That must have been the moment the bear finally decided we weren't worth messing around with.'

'What do you mean?' I ask.

'Well, it must have given him a terrible shock. Seals don't hit you round the head with a shovel!'

We both laugh.

'Thank God you were all right,' I say.

'Yes, I even managed to get some camera footage the first time it appeared.'

'Wow, I'd love to see it. Have you put it on YouTube?'

'I think it might be there,' she says.

'It is,' Sarah suddenly interjects. All this time I thought she'd been engrossed in what she was doing on her iPad and hadn't realised she'd been listening in on our conversation. 'But it's all wobbly,' she says disparagingly.

'I think we'll let your mum off for that,' I say. 'She was facing a polar bear, after all.'

'But do you know what?' Ann continues. 'Whilst I was terrified, that bear was one of the reasons I felt OK when I got pulled off the ice. I thought to myself: don't you dare spoil this, Ann, because you haven't got to the bloody pole. You've been on the most amazing adventure and you got to spend three days with a bear in its own habitat and neither of you got hurt. That bear has touched your life and you've touched his and now you've got that memory forever. I felt honoured,' she says. 'Really, really honoured.'

I notice immediately that she chooses the word D. H. Lawrence used when he met his snake. The same word I had felt when I was dropped into the deep waters of the Mediterranean in Formentera. For there is something extraordinarily special about encounters with the natural world at its most beautiful and dangerous. There is no better reminder of our insignificance and how lucky we all are to be on this glorious planet, whatever disappointments it brings our way.

At the end of our lunch, the word Ann gives me is 'privilege'. It was her privilege to face her polar bear, and it is my privilege to face the sea.

Then I turn to Sarah. 'Will you give me a word too?' I ask.

She looks at me and hesitates.

'Any word,' I say. 'There are no right ones and wrong ones. Choose any word you like.'

She hesitates again.

'"Can",' she says. 'You *can* swim the Channel.'

And what a wonderful word can is.

Where's the Manual?

The problem is, there's no definitive manual for training to swim the Channel. If there were I'd have bought it. It's not like running a marathon, where there are tried and tested formulas. Since Captain Webb first made it across in the late nineteenth century, fewer than 2,000 people have done it, most of them men. Land marathons, on the other hand, boast millions of participants. The New York City Marathon, reportedly the largest in the world, has over 50,000 runners every year, and the London Marathon isn't much smaller. And that's every year, not ever. In nearly 150 years, there have been only a couple of thousand Channel Swimmers *ever*.

Everyone I speak to has a different theory about what you need to do during winter training prior to the big swim of the summer. There's the distance camp, who say it's all about time in the water and recommend swimming a minimum of twenty-five kilometres a week. There's the speed camp, who say the winter is all about increasing your pace: they talk about doing '4 x 100-metre sprints off two minutes with fifteen seconds' rest'. Just the sound of this scares me.

I have no idea what it means and don't want to. And then there's the technique camp, who say that you need to focus on improving the physics of your stroke above all else. I was never good at physics (except the iron shavings and magnet test – who doesn't love that?) but after the shame of Coniston I know my stroke does need improvement. Nearly everyone says that during the winter getting into open water is pointless in training terms because it gets far colder than it will actually be when you swim so you can't stay in long enough. This means that you have to do the majority of your winter training in a pool.

For over a month I feel like I'm drowning in advice and I don't know what to do for the best. I want to hitch my boat to someone, but I don't know who to choose. It's creeping towards October and there is less than a year to go. Whenever I think this, I feel as if Munch's *The Scream* has been transposed into my head. I guess of all of them I prefer the advice of the technique camp, but maybe that's because it sounds the easiest? Maybe the testosterone-fuelled camps of speed and distance are what I need. I can sense my vacillation is starting to frustrate my advice-givers. They've got this look in their eyes that seems to say: *she doesn't have what it takes.* Boris sends me an email which reads: *'Jessica, you're going to have to hurt yourself in training every day from now until next summer if you want to stand a chance,'* and when I mention to Nick that I'm thinking of focusing on improving my stroke, he says bluntly that at some point (and I think he means this point) you've got to stop worrying about your technique and just start swimming. And Chris –

well, I haven't heard from Chris since Coniston, and I think that probably says a lot.

So I've made a decision. I'm going to write my own personalised Channel swimming manual. It's going to be based on what I've learned so far from other people, and what I know about myself which they don't. But please don't spread it around, because those who know about these things are bound to disagree. And if it works, well, I could patent it or something. So here it is . . .

Jessica's Channel Swimming Training Manual

1. Go back to swimming school to learn how to crawl.
2. Join a swimming club and attend once a week because there's nothing that makes you work harder than swimming with people who are faster than you (and nearly everyone in any swimming club is faster than me).
3. Do one speed session a week (shhh, only one, but that still means I'm going to have to learn the jargon).
4. Do one long swim a week, increasing my time by fifteen minutes each session, with the aim of reaching six hours in a pool by the spring so that I just have to repeat that in the sea to qualify.
5. Go to the Serpentine right the way through the winter even if it means I just get in for five minutes. I don't care that everybody says this is pointless: I've got to face down my fear of the cold.

6. Go to Formentera at the beginning of May next year with John and his team to do my six-hour qualifier (having already achieved six hours in the pool – see point 4).

7. Go down to Dover every weekend, from mid-May, and train with the other aspiring Channel swimmers who meet down there.

8. Join a gym with a pool so I can have a jacuzzi at the end of each session. It's all about the jacuzzi.

So there's the manual. My manual. I wonder why there isn't a manual for what happens when motherhood doesn't work either? There are manuals for how to get pregnant, and there are manuals for motherhood once you have. But there are no manuals for how to be a mother when you can't be a mother. Maybe after the Channel I'll have to write that manual as well.

The Ray, the Jellyfish and the Macrobiotic Mother

'Do you want to have a baby?'

I'm heading back to Formentera. It's not May yet (i.e. we've not reached point 6 of the manual), it's the beginning of October. John has organised a week of technique training and encouraged me to come along. He's promised me that the water's warm and there are no long swims on the agenda. I also have an ulterior motive for going, which I don't mention to anyone else. One of the many women who wrote to me after the 'no black tights' article has agreed to meet me for supper back on Ibiza island at the end of the week, just before I return to England. She's called Claudia and she's the one who wrote to me and said that she's in her mid-forties and has three children under the age of five, all of whom were conceived naturally (and none of them twins). She's English but lives in Spain, running regular fertility and mother and baby retreats on the island. I figure if there is anyone in the world who has the potential to persuade me that biological motherhood might still be a possibility post-forty-three, it's got to be her.

But first comes the sea. John's assistant, Alice, picks me up on my own from the ferry port as everyone else has already arrived.

'Don't worry,' she says. 'This week's going to be very different from the last one. And you haven't even met Ray yet.'

'What do you mean?'

'You'll see,' she says cryptically.

Ray is the special guest teacher for the week. I've been hearing his name for a while in swimming circles. He has a shed in Canary Wharf which houses an endless pool embedded with cameras. Here he films people's swimming stroke from all angles and coaches them on how to improve. John is visibly delighted that Ray's agreed to come to Formentera for the week to teach technique. Apparently, it's quite a coup. And when I meet Ray for the first time on the terrace of Can Rolls, I see exactly what Alice was talking about and why many people here will be delighted that Ray's come to teach technique too. He's got the looks and charisma of a mature male Hollywood star – he could be a contender for the next James Bond – and however good a swimming instructor he is, he's definitely wasted in a shed in Canary Wharf. For the rest of the week we all joke endlessly about having 'five minutes in the shallows with Ray'. It's not even wishful thinking, as we do all have regular sessions with him in the local pool and the sea, learning about extension, rotation and 'the catch', which refers to how your hands should be positioned as they move under the water. Ray says that he's seen plenty of dreadful swimmers cross the Channel through sheer bloody-mindedness and exertion, but if you get your stroke right you're going to be halfway there. It will mean that you go faster with less effort and reduce your risk of injury. I definitely like the idea of being halfway there before I've even got started, so I hang on to his every word.

By the end of the week, I've made an amendment to my Channel swimming manual. Point 1 now reads: 'Go back to swimming school *with Ray* to learn how to crawl.'

———————

On my last morning in Formentera, I decide to take a solitary swim at sunrise. Everyone else left yesterday, but because I'm staying on to have supper with Claudia in Ibiza this evening I stayed an extra night. The bay is calm, in darkness at first and then flooded with orange light as the sun emerges on the horizon. It's breathtakingly beautiful. I glide through the water, extending my arm purposefully with each stroke, just as Ray has taught us to do. But suddenly, as if an electric current has hit me, I let out an involuntary scream. It's happened. It's finally happened. I've met my Channel nemesis, and he's come all the way to Spain to greet me.

I stop swimming but my body continues to writhe in pain. I can't see my attacker but my back is stinging in a dozen places and I'm terrified it will want to say hello again. I start swimming breathlessly towards my towel, which I've left further along the beach, resorting back to the comfort of breaststroke. As soon as I get back to my room, I look at my back in the mirror to assess the damage. Whatever it was that stung me has left its mark. I'm covered in raised red welts which are throbbing with pain. But then I remember Ann Daniels and her polar bear and tell myself to (wo)man up. I'm alive; it was just a jellyfish.

As the morning progresses, the pain gradually subsides, and although there's no doubt I'll be water-weary for a while, I know I've just taken another important step in my Channel challenge. I've faced my own polar bear and survived.

———————

Claudia Spahr is the sort of woman who makes you want to turn the kitchen upside down in search of the juicer you got given for Christmas years ago and have never used. With a body honed by yoga and a macrobiotic diet, she belies her forty-six years. She's of Swiss German extraction, was bought up in Yorkshire and married a Spaniard, so not only has she had three children in her forties, they are also all trilingual – now that's showing off! In true Spanish style we arrange to meet late for drinks and tapas in Ibiza town. Nine-thirty is already approaching my preferred bedtime, and when she texts and postpones for an hour to 10:30, I have to consume a ton of caffeine to stay awake. I don't mention this when we meet; I'm not sure Claudia is the sort of woman who would approve of a double espresso.

We find a quiet café on a dimly lit backstreet with tables outside and order a couple of glasses of cava and a plate of prawns to share. I start by asking Claudia about her journey to motherhood: her children are now six, three and nearly one. Like many women she tells me she spent her twenties and thirties pursuing her career, partying and travelling the world, and she only met her husband when she was nearly forty. 'The thing is,' she says, 'I believe that women can carry on having babies right up until the menopause. It's only society that stops them. We're constantly being told that we have to have babies earlier and that if we do all the things that feminism gave us, we're risking our chance of becoming mothers. It's almost as if it's a conspiracy to keep women in their place.'

'Do you really think that?' I ask.

'Well, I do think that older motherhood is one of the last taboos. No one thinks twice about interracial couples or gay couples having children these days. But put a grandmother with a pregnant belly on the front cover of a magazine and it's designed to shock us.'

There are a lot of eminent medical professionals who wouldn't agree with Claudia's theory about being able to get pregnant right up to menopause. Although some women do fall pregnant naturally in their late forties and even fifties, it's pretty unusual, and the dangers to mother and baby are increased. I remember when Cherie Blair did. The world was shocked, and not just because of her age (forty-seven) but because we had to get our heads round the fact that she and the prime minister still had sex despite their busy schedules. Of course lots of celebrities manage it, but the little discussed fact is that the majority of 'post-forty-three' celebrity births are the result of egg donation from a younger woman.

But where I do think Claudia is definitely right is that, unless you're a celebrity, older motherhood is still regarded as a bit distasteful, though society doesn't seem to have a problem with older fatherhood. In fact, celebrity men can continue fathering babies into their dotage without anyone raising an eyebrow. Most of the Rolling Stones are still at it. I know that societal opinion is part of my dilemma about what to do next in my pursuit of motherhood. Even if I could become a mother approaching my mid-forties, I'm now also worried about being considered a freak.

'So you really believe as long as a woman's having periods nature intends for her to conceive?' I ask.

'I do.'

'But what about the IVF statistics which show that success rates drop so significantly after forty?'

'Yes, but the average age of first-time mothers is increasing and what we don't know is what would have happened if IVF hadn't been invented.'

She's right. IVF has definitely upset the natural fertility ecosystem. Who knows how many couples have turned to clinical intervention, without it being really necessary, because of the constant scaremongering women in their thirties have to face that they might have left it too late? And what if all the fertility drugs that get pumped into your system when you're going through treatment end up hindering rather than helping your fertility? I try not to think about what I've injected into myself over the years.

'So,' I say. 'What would your advice be?'

'About what?'

'To me? Do you really think I can still have my own biological baby even after everything I've been through?'

'Actually, I can't tell whether you want to have a baby,' says Claudia.

I'm totally taken aback by her answer. It definitely wasn't the one I was expecting. 'I've read the stuff you've written,' she continues, 'and you're very funny about what you've been through, but it seems to me it obscures what you really think. Do you *want* to have a baby?'

I'm silent for a while, taking in the enormity of what she's just said. She watches me carefully.

I take a breath of the Spanish night air before responding: 'I think ... I think that despite everything you've been saying, I won't be able to make it happen.'

'You mean you don't trust your body any more?' she says. 'I'm not surprised: IVF does that to you.'

'It's more than that,' I reply. 'I think I don't trust that I should be a mother.'

'But that's just about confidence,' Claudia says. 'For a long time no one believed anyone could swim the Channel, and then they did.'

———

The next morning when I go down to breakfast in my hotel I think about my conversation with Claudia. Had all the years we'd spent trying to conceive and all the repeated IVF failures resulted in me losing confidence not only in becoming pregnant but in being a mother at all? And although I still wasn't sure whether I was capable of swimming the Channel either, the fact that I had survived my first jellyfish attack had injected me with a confidence that I didn't have last week. So I decide to order fresh fruit salad for breakfast – it's possibly the most colour my intestines have seen in months – and as the word Claudia had given me for my swim was 'water', I have that instead of a coffee. I hope the macrobiotic mother would be proud.

VO2 Max

I've joined a gym. It's not the first time but it is the first time in a long time. The pool there is only twenty-one metres long and next to a rather nice steam room, sauna and jacuzzi. These are definitely not Channel conditions – I spend most of the time pushing off the side and sometimes the place is pleasantly steaming, like a jungle. As a new member, the club offer me a free health MOT and I decide to book myself an appointment. A gym guy – tall, black, rippling muscles – leads me to a little windowless room in the basement. He asks me about my health goals and I tell him about the Channel. He seems impressed. We go through the initial questions about hereditary illnesses, operations, medications, etc. My answer is a continual 'no' because I don't suppose a decade of unsuccessful fertility treatment counts in these sorts of questionnaires.

Then gym guy says, embarrassed: 'I always hate this next question . . . Are you pregnant?'

I think about all that that question holds. At least people are still asking it. One day soon surely they'll stop.

We then move on to alcohol consumption. I love drinking

almost as much as I love eating, but trying for a baby has gradually ruined our beautiful relationship. For a long time now our dealings have become uneasy, tinged with guilt and suspicion, as it's one of the first things you are advised to give up if you want to conceive. I've tried not drinking. I've tried controlling someone else's drinking. And when neither of those things resulted in a baby, I tried to drink normally again. I tried not to think about drinking – mine or anyone else's. But I still did because when you can't get pregnant, you can't stop shaping your life around anything that might make a difference, even if it doesn't.

'Maybe about ten units,' I say.

'Ten!?' gym guy says. He looks shocked.

'Well, you know, whatever the recommended weekly units are, it's under that. I'm allowed fourteen, aren't I?'

I wonder whether I should say there's hardly a risk of me getting pregnant or anything, although I don't.

'But you're training to swim the Channel,' gym guy reprimands.

'So?'

'You can't drink if you're training for something like that.'

'Well, last week I drank hardly anything at all,' I counter defensively.

'What did you have?' he challenges me.

I think back. Two glasses of red wine with Sunday lunch and a glass of Madeira on Friday night. The Madeira had been a mistake.

'Maybe about five units,' I say confidently.

'Over how many days?'

'About three,' I say, less so.

OK, technically, it was two days. But you need to be on your guard with these how-many-units questions. I'd like to know who enjoys a drink and is able to answer them honestly. Dinner for two with a bottle of wine and you're veering rapidly towards your weekly limit. And who sets the figures anyway? They're different in every country. If I lived on the other side of the Channel I would be officially allowed more units than over here. I stop. I'm starting to think and sound like someone else who is not supposed to be in this story.

'Fine,' says gym guy, sensing the sensitivity of the subject. 'On to the next bit. Weight and height.'

'Oh God,' I say.

'Yes, sorry, women always hate this bit.'

'Actually, I'm supposed to be putting on weight,' I tell him.

He looks as if he doesn't quite believe me before asking why. I explain about the cold as he measures me against the wall before declaring me five foot eight. I step on the scales. I know this isn't going to be good. I put on my 'no black tights' red dress last week – the first time in several months – and it was snug. I know that under the circumstances this is supposed to be a good thing but it is also a very bad thing. You can't wipe out years of being body-conscious even if you are training to swim the Channel.

'That looks like 10 stone 8.' He pauses for a second. 'No, sorry, 10 stone 10.'

My stomach lurches: 10 stone 10! 'It's probably the hood,' I say in explanation.

Gym guy looks at me, confused.

'I knew I shouldn't have worn the top with the hood. I reckon hoods like these weigh at least as much as a couple of bags of sugar.'

His confusion turns to bewilderment. 'Ten stone 10 is fine at your height,' he says.

'Not if your aim in life is to be under ten stone.'

'But I thought you said you were trying to put on weight for the swim.'

'Yeah, well, I am. But it's too early for ten pounds. It would be fine if I were doing it next week, but there are still ten months to go.'

'Well, let's test your blood pressure then,' gym guy says, clearly trying to change the subject. He straps the band to my left arm. Systolic is 112, diastolic is 73 and my resting heart rate is 52, which he says bodes well for my 'VO2 max' – whatever that is. We carry on with the tests. Blood glucose levels are fine but the cholesterol is slightly elevated. I ask whether it could have anything to do with the two packets of crisps I had just before I arrived (note, they were small ones). Gym guy says it's possible but unlikely.

And so to the VO2 max test itself, which apparently measures your aerobic fitness and is an important determinant of your endurance during prolonged exercise. I need this to be good. He gets me to strap a little box to my chest, then lies me down on an examination couch and gently places what looks like a stopwatch above it. I lie there for a long time focusing on my breathing and trying to work out what might lead to a successful result. I don't want to mess this one up. I need it to be better than the alcohol, the cholesterol and the scales. After what seems like an inordinately long time, the stopwatch beeps and gym guy retrieves it.

'I knew it,' he says excitedly. 'Your VO2 max is excellent.'

'It is?' I say, surprised.

'Yes, it's forty-two. That's in the elite category for your age.'

'Are you sure you put the right age in?'

'Twenty-first of November, 1970, right?'

'Yeah, no need to say it out loud,' I say quickly.

Gym guy laughs.

'So, now for the moment of truth – your total fitness score,' he says, building the suspense as if we're on a TV talent show.

I wish he'd told me this was a proper test; I reckon I could have scored better on some of the earlier questions if I'd known. Like the water question. I bet the 'how many glasses of water do you drink a day' question has let me down. I'm good with drinking enough alcohol but dreadful with water.

'And your score is . . . 740 out of 1,000,' gym guy says. 'That's great.'

'Really?' I say. I sound surprised. For years now, I've been so used to my body letting me down, and my mind berating me for its inadequacy.

'So what do I need to do to improve my fitness even further?' I ask.

'You don't need to anything,' gym guy replies. 'I wish my

VO2 was elite, although it does say here you should drink more water.'

'These days, I spend my life in it. Doesn't that count?'

The Internet Entrepreneur

'I think life could absolutely be fulfilling without children ...
The tragedy is when people don't think it can be.'

'So what did you want to be when you were a little girl?'

'I wanted to be Kevin Keegan,' she says.

I laugh.

'Did motherhood figure?'

'I didn't view myself as particularly maternal. I was a tomboy, obsessed with football in an age where there weren't really ladettes. I'm a lifelong Liverpool fan.'

'So if you had to choose between motherhood and football, which would one would win?'

It seems bizarre that my conversation with the woman who has defined the voice of the modern mother starts on a topic that is synonymous with men and blokeishness. Justine Roberts is the founder of Mumsnet, the biggest and most influential internet site for mothers in the UK. In fact, it's so influential that it has been credited with determining the outcome of general elections. She has agreed to meet me one morning at what she describes as 'Mumsnet Towers', the company's headquarters.

I decide I'm going to bring muffins – for me there's no more iconic representation of motherhood in a breakfast cake. But en route to meet her, I discover my favourite muffin shop, Muffinski's, has closed down. This is both a short- and long-term disaster and sends me into a flurry. What can I bring instead? In a panic, I decide on doughnuts. It's not muffins but it will do, although I have to go to Sainsbury's to get them because I recently had a doughnut disaster too. For years, I'd always buy them from Patisserie Valerie as they did the best cream doughnuts ever. Many of my teenage traumas were talked out in the original café on Soho's Old Compton Street in swirling smoke, back in the days when cigarettes were allowed. But then, around about the time the chain started to expand, they went and changed doughnut supplier and the new ones aren't half as nice. Peter wrote to them to complain and, although I'm not allowed to mention him, I know he won't mind me telling you that because it's a matter of principle. He's a doughnut vigilante.

Justine laughs at my question and then tells me that her version of motherhood is so intrinsically tied up with football she doesn't need to choose. She's nuts about it; her kids are nuts about it. Everyone enjoys watching and playing. So, I ask – given she'd never thought of herself as maternal – what was the turning point?

'Well, although I didn't think about it, I suppose I always thought I would become a mother,' she says. 'I just thought, that will be what will happen when it happens. My partner and I met at university and we were together for quite a long time before we got married, and if you ask why we got married it was probably because we thought we might be thinking about having children, but it was never articulated like that.'

'And then after you got married did it happen quickly?'

'Yes, I got pregnant immediately and had twins, and they were ten weeks premature, so in actual fact I had children seven and half months after first deciding we might try.'

'And you've got four now, haven't you? Did you always know you wanted a big family?'

'No. I've always been quite passive, which I know seems contrary to who I am at work. My husband did though. He was an only child until he was ten and was very conscious he wanted a gang. I was less certain but fairly . . .' She thinks for a moment about what word to use and then chooses 'haphazard' and laughs at her choice. 'So we ended up with a gang.'

As I listen to Justine's relaxed attitude to having children – it will happen when it happens – and then that she fell pregnant straight away, I feel a tightening in my chest. Justine is only three years older than me and in what feels like some sort of cruel coincidence I'd read this morning before coming here that she was at New College, Oxford, which was where I had applied to go to university but didn't get in as my A-level results weren't good enough. Now I find out that, like me, she never focused on motherhood in her twenties and just assumed it would happen. For her it did. She's even got a gang. I've always wanted four children too because, like Justine's husband, I essentially grew up as an only child. (I have a sister who is ten years older than me from my mum's first marriage, but she left home to live with her boyfriend when I was only six.) And if all that wasn't enough, Justine Roberts has also created a hugely successful business; Radio 4 says she's the seventh most influential woman in the UK. She's even recently launched a new website called Gransnet, which I'm probably never going to be eligible to use either. I don't want to but, by comparison, I can't help but feel like a failure.

The Nobel Prize-winning psychologist Daniel Kahneman has said that there are two types of envy: good envy and bad envy. Good envy can be motivating; it can make you work hard to get what you want. Bad envy is dangerously destructive and is at its most potent when you're comparing yourself to someone who is close or similar to you and has achieved more. That's when envy, he says, becomes 'true pain'.* It's not Justine's fault that I'm finding our meeting hard. She's given up time in her incredibly busy schedule to see me and she's being generous with her responses to my crazy questions. It's just that bad envy has decided to come with me and my doughnuts to Mumsnet Towers to meet her.

I look at my laptop and dare myself to ask her what she thinks would have happened if she hadn't been able to have children. She tells me honestly that she hasn't ever really thought about it, but clearly her life would have been

---

* Daniel Kahneman, *The Why Factor: Envy*, BBC World Service, 31 March 2014

different, and she wouldn't have started Mumsnet. 'I do sometimes have those moments where I'm slightly envious of people who haven't got the chaos,' she says. 'People who have beautiful houses with lots of cream and beige.'

Her words catch me for a moment. Could Justine Roberts be envious of me? No, there isn't any cream and beige in my house, just grey.

I start to ask her whether she thinks a life without children could ever be as fulfilling and before I finish my sentence, she cuts in: 'I think life could absolutely be fulfilling without children. I really genuinely believe that. The tragedy is when people don't think it can be. That's the thing that will stop it.' There is such passion and persuasion in her voice that I want to believe her. She continues: 'There are so many wonderful relationships you can have with people. In fact, one of the things I feel guilty about is that I have very little time for my friends and some of them have very little time for me. People you love and care about but you forget their birthdays, you don't speak to them for months on end. But there are all kinds of relationships that are tremendously fulfilling.'

I know there is something important in what Justine's just said, but I'm going to need time to process it. Having children can be a very effective shortcut to building a close relationship with another human being, but maybe she's right, it's not the only meaningful relationship you can have. Would it be possible to replace the parent–child bond with other sorts of relationships that might actually be its equal?

Our conversation feels so important and sincere that it

emboldens me to ask her whether she feels that the rise of Mumsnet has been divisive for women, creating a sense of the haves and the have-nots. I know it's a tricky question because any good business segments the market, and her market is mums. She acknowledges it happens and says it's partly to do with the way the media positions motherhood as a mythical, almost virginal, state, which has elevated the mother's voice against the non-mother's voice. But then she adds that this is a double-edged sword, as it sometimes means mothers are also portrayed as insular and stupid. She says it disappoints her that there isn't a powerful and obvious equivalent to Mumsnet for women who are not mothers, because what's most important is that women's voices get heard. Again, her observation is carefully considered and shingle-sharp, but I can't help wishing Justine had founded 'Womensnet' instead. The truth is, I don't want to listen to the voice of the 'non-mother'; it's not a voice I ever wanted to be. In fact, ironically, I've probably tried harder and thought more about being a mother than most mothers ever have. Mumsnet should be in my browser history, not Fertility Friends. I say this to Justine, but I don't mention that I feel she might actually be living my life; that would be too weird.

'To be fair, you could have that dialogue on Mumsnet,' she says. 'You don't have to identify or anything. No one's checking your credentials at the door. And besides, the bulk of the conversation is not about motherhood, it's about life. It's about my boss, my partner, my mother-in-law, my neighbours. Am I right to feel what I feel about those things? Am I right to think that *Downton Abbey* was rubbish last night? Our biggest forum is: am I being unreasonable? It's massively bigger than anything on pregnancy or parenting or sleep. And it's mostly about people's relationships with their partners.'

'Maybe,' I say, pondering what's she said. 'I still think I would feel a bit of a fraud going on it.' I then confess that I'd once seriously considered going to a pregnancy yoga class. It's something I've always looked forward to and I figured I could just go along and pretend and no one would know. I thought this might amuse her because I'd read she practises yoga regularly. She laughs and says: 'Don't worry, it's not that much fun because you can't do anything!'

———

Later, after my meeting with Justine, I go onto the Mumsnet homepage and scroll through all the topics. It's the end of October and there's a picture of two children stamping through autumn leaves in a park and the words: 'Everything you need for a stress-free half-term.' And next to this: 'Brilliant last-minute costumes for Halloween,' and then: 'Avoid the Christmas panic – this year's most wanted toys.' And below this there are features on 'Bedtime', 'Potty training' and 'Nailing the working mum routine'. I close the window. I want to engage, but I can't. I have no costumes to make or toys to buy, and the only routine I have to juggle is fitting in work with swimming training. Maybe somewhere behind this, if I were brave enough to look, there would be conversations on the latest episode of *Downton Abbey*. But I'm not brave enough.

I think back to the moment we said goodbye in her office. My box of doughnuts had sat on the table untouched throughout our conversation. She kindly offered me one to take with me and I accepted, but she didn't take one herself. I suspect my internet entrepreneur doesn't eat many doughnuts. Justine Roberts is beautifully slim. Correction. Justine Roberts is beautifully *thin*. There is no slow slide to the voluptuous going on with her.

There it is again – true pain.

The word she gave me was 'grit'.

Where is it, Jessica? Where is your bloody grit?

Odi et Amo

It's always bemused me that I took ancient history and Latin at A level, along with English, which I went on to study at university (Leeds, not Oxford). I'm hopeless at foreign languages and Latin isn't even one you can use. And I still have trouble remembering who came first, the Romans or the Greeks. When I chose Sappho as the first woman on my list of twenty-one, I had to check which she was. She's Greek. That means she came before the Romans.

Thinking back, it was, in fact, my school classics teacher, Mr Buckley, not me, who was responsible for my A-level choices. He was one of the very best teachers in school. Everybody loved him, and consequently, everybody loved Latin, which, in hindsight, was a rather remarkable thing in an inner London comprehensive which took girls from all backgrounds and academic abilities. He wasn't even conventionally handsome. He was small, rotund and ginger, but his enthusiasm for his subject radiated around the classroom. It just goes to show how important good teachers are, and although it's a brilliant line, I hate George Bernard Shaw for writing, 'Those who can, do; those who can't, teach', because its denigration of the teaching profession is reprehensible. And Woody Allen didn't help when he riffed on the line and said: 'Those who can't do, teach, and those who can't teach, teach gym.' He obviously never had Ray teach him swimming.

But just after I made the decision to take Latin and ancient history as my A levels, Mr Buckley went and committed the ultimate betrayal and got a new job in a posh private school. I've never quite forgiven him. He left us with a teacher who wasn't half as good, and my interest in these subjects quickly waned. I got an A in English (thanks to another great teacher) and, although I did pass the other two, let's just say I cried when I got the results, and they weren't tears of joy.

I will always thank Mr Buckley for one thing though. He left me a two-line legacy in Latin that has stayed with me throughout my life.

> *Odi et amo, quare id faciam fortasse requiris?*
> *Nescio sed fieri sentio et excrucior.*

These are the words of the Roman poet, Catullus, to his mistress, Lesbia. Just two lines that say more to me than the 9,896 lines of Virgil's *Aeneid* ever will.

> *I hate and I love. Why do I do it, perhaps you ask?*
> *I do not know, but I feel it happen and I am tortured by it.*

I find it extraordinary that a twenty-something man who

was alive more than 2,000 years ago can articulate so exactly what I, as a forty-something woman, feel today. And I'm not talking about my meeting with Justine Roberts or about swimming – at least not only about them. I'm talking about the silence in this story. The person who has been with me since the beginning of my pursuit of motherhood, but now as I try to reach the end seems to be slipping away. I don't know what has happened to us but I know something has. I hate and I love, and I am tortured by it.

The Businesswoman

'Grief can drive you apart.'

The woman I meet after internet entrepreneur Justine Roberts is Nicola Horlick, the original icon of superwomanhood, and I fear I may be heading towards my nadir.

After graduating from university (Oxford), Nicola Horlick went into the City, saved a bank and got paid extremely well for it. But it wasn't until she had a spectacular public falling out with her employer that anyone really knew who she was. In the furore that ensued the press discovered that, as well as being a formidable financier, she was also a mother of five (later to become six). With this she was catapulted to the pinnacle of feminist success, the media coining her 'the woman who has it all'. Now, like Martin Luther King Jr, who will forever be dreaming, and Catherine Tate, who will never be bovvered, Nicola Horlick will always be the woman who is having it all.

So when I wrote my list of people that I wanted to meet Nicola Horlick was near the top. There seemed no one better to ask what had given most fulfilment: a high-flying career or motherhood. I was conscious, however, that I would need to pose the question very carefully, because in 1998, Nicola lost her twelve-year-old daughter, Georgie, after a long battle with leukaemia.

But when the day of our meeting finally comes there is something else I want to ask her, a new question that a few months ago, when I first started my list, might not have even been a consideration. I would have to pose this question cautiously too – I wasn't yet sure whether I'd dare.

'Does it make you cross?' I ask when we meet at her offices in Mayfair. We're sitting in a beautiful room on two canary yellow chairs, light flooding in from north- and south-facing windows. There's no table so I'm balancing a cup of coffee on my knee. Nicola doesn't drink coffee, she tells me. Or tea. Maybe that's why she doesn't need a table. Between us on the floor is an unopened box of macaroons that I've bought from the French patisserie Ladurée, in Burlington Arcade. Macaroons for Mayfair – I figured it was apt.

'The having-it-all thing drives me completely crazy,' she says. 'Today is actually the sixteenth anniversary of my daughter's death. And it makes me so angry when people say that I'm the woman who has it all, because obviously I'd much rather have Georgie than a successful career, money and everything else.'

So I ask, curious, what her career has given her versus motherhood. She tells me that having a successful career has definitely been fulfilling, and latterly she's set up her own business, which has been even more rewarding than working for a huge nebulous organisation, although also extremely stressful because you don't have a big bank behind you. Motherhood has been massively fulfilling too, she says, and she feels incredibly lucky but also incredibly unlucky because, although a Victorian mother would probably have had seven children and three would have died, today in the Western world, child death is extremely rare.

It's only at this point that I notice that she's wearing a lot of black, and I wonder whether it has anything to do with the importance of the day. It seems significant to me that that this is the day we finally meet.

Then, with my encouragement, Nicola starts to talk about all her children. She enthusiastically tells me their names, ages, birthdays, what they're doing, where they're living, details of their girlfriends and boyfriends, the challenges they've faced and their impressive achievements. She's obviously deeply engaged with their lives and her pride in them feels like it somehow spurs her. But I can't help wondering: why, when she has such a demanding career, did she choose to have quite so many children?

Almost as if she senses my train of thought, she says suddenly: 'The thing is, when I was a child, if I had to make a wish, I'd always wish that my mother had another child because there was only me and my brother. I thought that was incredibly dull, and I really desperately wanted siblings. So I think I would always have had more than two children. But I was aiming for four. I ended up having six because of Georgie being sick. When she got this dreadful thing called fasciitis and nearly died, I had this desperate desire to have more and got pregnant just after that. And then when she died, I had this desperate need to have another baby. So I did and he was very, very comforting. It was good that I had him. Definitely.'

I'm struck by the number of times she says the word 'desperate', with its sense of urgency and fear, and by her use of the word 'definitely' in affirmation. I suddenly realise that her answer has shone what might be a light.

'Nicola,' I ask, 'are you someone who is afraid to be alone?'

She pauses, just for a moment, but it's possibly the first time she's paused at any of my questions – her answers are so fluid and articulate. 'I used to hate being alone,' she says. 'But now I quite like it.' She pauses again and then qualifies her answer. 'Sometimes.'

'But what if all your family were away and you were faced with the prospect of a week with no one around. Would that terrify you a bit?'

'I've only slept in the house once on my own. I remember feeling slightly anxious. I'm not neurotic in any way but I imagined that people with knives were going to break in and stab me.' She continues in explanation: 'You see, I got mugged outside our house.' Her words quicken. 'It hasn't really affected me at all, I never really think about it, but if I was alone I would probably lock the shutters.' Her answer confuses me; maybe my question wasn't clear. It wasn't really about the danger of burglars in the night; it was about the terror of being alone in the world without anyone to love and need you. That, for me, is one of the most frightening things about childlessness: the eternal loneliness. But there is suddenly something about the truth of our exchange, even in its opacity, that gives me the confidence to ask my other question, the one I wasn't sure if I'd dare to ask.

When preparing for my meeting with Nicola today I listened to a radio interview that she had done seventeen years ago. It had been recorded just prior to her daughter's death and the interviewing psychiatrist, Professor Anthony Clare, had asked about the pressures that Georgie's illness had put on her relationship with her husband. Nicola had answered simply that if you have a good relationship it gets stronger and if you have a bad relationship it breaks down, and that she was fortunate to have a good relationship. But a few years after her daughter's death, she and her husband divorced, and I hoped I might find the opportunity to ask her about it.

'Please don't feel like you have to answer this if it's too personal,' I say tentatively, 'but I wonder if you could tell me why your first marriage ended?' She doesn't close me down, so I continue: 'I ask because for the past couple of months my partner and I have been struggling. Really struggling. People always say that our relationship must be such a good one because of what we've been through together, but now I don't know. It's frightening.'

'Grief can drive you apart,' she says.

'Didn't you once say it made you stronger?'

'In our case, what I found was that when Georgie was sick we were very much bonded together. Our lives were driven by what the doctors were telling us and we went up and down emotionally together. But then when she actually died, it was different. My husband found it really difficult and I think every time he looked at me when he woke up in the morning it just reminded him of the terrible loss. He couldn't cope with that at all. But rather than saying so, he just started doing stupid things.'

'Like what?' I ask.

I am shocked by the candour and private detail of her response but try not to show it.

'I tried really hard for two years to hold it together,' she says. 'In the end I just couldn't. I said to him, I felt as though I had been dangling over a precipice with two ropes holding me up. One had been cut when Georgie died and I was now like this' – she lifts her arms in the air and then drops one to show me what she means. 'And then when the rope that was my marriage was cut, I fell into this abyss. I became seriously clinically depressed.'

'So what happened?'

'I went to a psychiatrist who tried to put me on medication and have me hospitalised. But I wanted to get through it on my own and somehow I did. I don't know how because I actually honestly wanted to die. I thought my life wasn't worth living.' She stops in thought for a few moments: 'I've never told anyone that.'

We both feel the force of her revelation. It hangs in the air between us like the rope that was cut and which left her falling, and then she says: 'Although I don't know about your situation, I imagine it's a bit like grief: you are probably grieving for the baby you haven't had. And so's he. You may feel there's nothing to hold you together if there isn't a child.'

Again her words hang between us, heavy and horrible, bringing into focus that I'm not just sitting with a woman who knows what it is to have lost a child but also a woman who knows what it is to have lost a relationship that might never have been lost if it hadn't been for that first loss. A woman who has experienced loss upon loss, and who surely knows at the deepest level what it feels like to be alone, and how frightening that is.

The magnitude of the moment is broken by the sound of someone on the stairs outside. Nicola's PA comes in.

'Your next appointment is here,' she says – my cue to wrap up.

I put down my half-drunk cup of coffee on the floor. 'I've just got one more very quick question,' I say as I start to gather my things and put on my coat.

The word she gives me is 'strength'.

The Solitude of Swimming

In the pool today, on my forty-fourth birthday, I spent 110 lengths wondering how you write about someone and something that you're not supposed to be writing about. Has grief driven us apart? Or was it holding us together in the first place? I'm not entirely sure what's happened, but I know something has. I feel us disappearing from one another. I can't hold on as tight any more.

Was I was naive to think that this new journey I've embarked on was somehow our journey, like the last one we travelled together? How could it be, with all these hours in the pool alone? There is nothing more solitary than swimming. Has my longed-for redemption become just another way of redoubling my pain? Because, like Nicola Horlick – the woman who doesn't have it all – I harbour a fundamental fear of being alone: of dying without my children by my side, of a funeral with no one there. Yet I thought that there would always be you, and now I don't know. In the end, like the solitude of swimming, perhaps we all have to come to terms with our fundamental aloneness in the world.

I can feel tears in my goggles but here in the pool no one knows, not even the water, because water only knows tears as itself. I'm at a loss what to do so I keep swimming, silently counting the lengths.

The Filmmaker

Dear Jessica,

Thanks for your email. It all sounds really interesting but I had a baby at a chaotic time of my life and it was a very bad thing for me. I've never had maternal longings – they're a complete mystery to me – I also think we should be more supportive to people who decide not to have children and that there are too many people in the world.

Good luck with everything, dear Jessica.

Love Kim x

The Filmmaker, Part II

'You have to be happy with who you are . . .
You've got to find your people.'

What sort of self-respecting would-be endurance athlete would leave it that? She sounds exactly like the sort of person I need to meet. So I write back to the documentary filmmaker, Kim Longinotto, and tell her how valuable her perspective will be. I'm delighted when she concedes, and invites me round to her house for a cup of tea.

I decide to take a red velvet cake from an artisan bakery chain as my edible offering. It seems a seasonal choice given that it's just before Christmas. This is the first time anyone I've written to has invited me into their home, and I am immediately struck that the woman who says she has no maternal longings lives in a house with the sort of familial atmosphere that I have always dreamed of living in. There aren't any children in evidence, or a Christmas tree laden with presents. But during the three hours I spend in her large, open-plan kitchen the comings and goings of friends, lodgers and neighbours generate a conviviality that contrasts starkly to our own small, increasingly silent, flat.

I'm pretty sure it's significant that the first thing we talk about is Kim's mother. Kim tells me how relieved she was when she died. Her first ever memory, at two years old, before she could even really talk, was standing in the bathroom at home thinking she didn't like either of her parents but knowing that this was a terrible secret that she would have to keep to herself. When she tells me this, I ask whether she thinks her relationship to motherhood has been defined by her relationship with her own mother. But Kim says she believes they are only vaguely connected and that she's pretty sure she'd have felt the same if they hadn't had the relationship they did. Then, as if she's processing what I've said, she says, 'But maybe I wouldn't. In which case I'm glad I had the mother I had, because I'm happy . . . you have to be happy with who you are.'

At this point one of the inhabitants of the house comes in and we stop talking about motherhood and start talking about the cake. Kim knows the man who made it – not literally, but she knows the man who set up the bakery where I bought it. She tells me he wanted to be a filmmaker but ended up baking cakes instead. It was probably a wise move: it's definitely easier getting a cake into production than a film. This is one of the things I find impressive about Kim: she's become very successful in a highly competitive, male-dominated world, but despite her views on motherhood it's clear she's not done it by becoming some sort of pseudo-masculine stereotype. She's beguilingly feminine, so this sheds no light on her views on motherhood either.

'Do you make cakes?' the man who has joined us in the

kitchen asks me, coming over to cut himself a slice. I've already had one slice but Kim hasn't taken any yet, even though she is clearly delighted by the cake's presence.

'I have been known to,' I say (although I haven't attempted anything since the banana bread). 'One good thing about swimming the Channel is it's a licence to eat cake.'

'When are you doing it?' Kim asks.

'In the summer. If I'm up to it.'

'Are you practising?'

'A lot. I'm even going to swim in the Serpentine in Hyde Park on Christmas Day.'

Kim makes a sound of horror mixed with admiration, which is kind of how I feel about it too. And then we're alone again, minus a man and a slice of cake, and our motherhood conversation continues. I tell her about some of the other women I've met so far.

'What is Mumsnet?' Kim asks innocently when I mention Justine Roberts.

I explain that it's a website phenomenon that has galvanised the mummy voice.

'Well, I hate the mummy voice,' Kim says. 'When people say "as a parent" they're always going to say something really reactionary, like "as a parent we need our SUVs to take the kids to school". What happens to people with kids is all that matters is the kid and all their politics and everything goes.' She pauses mid-flow before repeating the word 'Mumsnet' and adding: 'even the name makes me feel ill.'

The funny thing, though, is that whilst Kim is definitively derogatory about the concept of mummyhood, she is clearly captivated by alternative parenting stories, going on to tell me at length about a newspaper article she's recently read about a family with thirty-four children – twenty-nine of them adopted – and about friends of hers, a lesbian couple, who adopted a little girl from an orphanage in China; she had been a victim of the country's one-child policy.

'What I can't bear,' she says when I ask about her fascination with these stories, 'and, Jessica, I'll just be honest with you, and it's not an attack on you or anything, but it's this idea of your own biological child: that it's yours and it belongs to you. It's the root of a lot of evils in the world; it's what's led to female genital mutilation and chastity belts and this obsession with women being pure. Because the link to that is that the men need to know that the child is theirs. So they do all these extraordinary things like veiling women, cutting them and now shooting them so they don't go to school. When you trace it back, the justification of it is this: how will you know that the children are yours if you don't? Because people feel like they get their immortality from their children: it's their legacy, it's them. That's why the man has to give the name. And even people I know who are really cool are obsessed with family trees and their name and all that. The older I live and the more films I make, the more I hate this motherhood thing. And fatherhood thing. It's such a trap. That's why I love people who have adopted because they've broken out of that totally and they've given a new life for a kid and love the children as their own.'

Kim specialises in making films about women who have been marginalised and oppressed. She knows more than most what that means, and her words make me think again of that phrase: *genetic imperialism*. But then I think of me and Molly and of healing the pain. Are these things different, or are they the same? I venture that it's strange and possibly controversial that Kim has these feelings as a biological mother herself.

'It makes it totally controversial, and people are quite shocked. But then I shock people all the time,' she says, batting it away until I ask how. 'On everything really,' she says. 'I tend to say things straight and then it upsets people. I've upset *Newsnight*, I've upset *Woman's Hour*...' Her voice trails off as if there's a longer list but something specific has come into her mind, and then she proceeds to tell me that last Christmas Eve she was interviewed on Radio 4's *Woman's Hour* about her latest film, and at the end of the show the presenter had said: 'Well, have a lovely Christmas, Kim, I hope you've got lots of bubbly wine in.' To which Kim replied: 'Actually, I don't really drink, but I do like a spliff.' And because the show was live, the presenter had an apoplectic fit, gesticulating at her silently but wildly to 'cut' by slashing an imaginary knife across her neck. But Kim was indignant and said on air that she'd just had to sit and listen for ages to a piece on sherry and she was just being honest. When she was taken to the green room afterwards, she was told she probably wouldn't be invited back. If that were me – and you know how I feel about Radio 4 – I'd probably have berated myself for most of the following year, but something tells me that Kim is the sort of woman who doesn't care. She's not going to say the right thing because it would be good for her career. And she's not going to say the right thing about motherhood because she's a mother. She's going to say what she thinks when she thinks it. It's a high-risk strategy for life but it's one that can gain you a lot of respect if it works, and in just over an hour she's gained mine.

I'm conscious, however, that we haven't yet touched at all on her own motherhood story, so I ask her if she's ready to tell it and it plays like a movie. A young, beautiful woman; an older, controlling man; sex, secrets and subterfuge. And then a baby, unwanted yet loved, but perhaps not enough. Because for Kim making films is clearly everything; telling other people's stories seems to be more important to her than living her own. She confesses that when she was making a film about night workers she would even leave her baby son alone to go off and film, coming back in the morning to him crying.

'You came home and he was crying?' I ask, trying to hide my disbelief.

'Yes, for ages, and I felt really bad. But, you see, Jessica, I feel quite strongly about one thing.' I've noticed that when she wants to emphasise something she addresses me directly. 'And I know this is right. I think there's a terrible blackmail that our society does, and all societies do, that you can't talk honestly about your attitude to childhood and to motherhood because it's a person.'

She's right. It's difficult for a child to say it doesn't love its mother, and perhaps even harder for a mother to say she doesn't love her child. And even though it's clear that Kim loves her son as a person, and from what she tells me about him he clearly loves her, this didn't make her *want* to be a mother. Motherhood is not every woman's calling or even every mother's calling. Sometimes children can be loved but unwanted. And sometimes unwanted children can be better loved elsewhere, if you're prepared to dig up and set fire to the family tree.

We are coming to the end of our conversation.

'What's happiness to you, Kim?' I ask.

'Being with people you love, and having a really good laugh,' she says. 'The best times I've had have been outside with friends,' and then she adds mischievously, 'with a spliff. I mean you don't need the spliff, it's just the spliff seems to somehow . . .' She breaks off and then says in a non sequitur: 'Did you see the film *Boyhood*?' I nod. 'God, that film's got a brilliant end. They're out on the canyon, and they've taken some dope, and he says, "I'm totally in the moment." And she says, "You're not in the moment, the moment's in you." And those are the moments when I'm happiest; when you know you're in the moment. You probably don't remember it because you're not a druggy like me, but that's a real stoner comment.'

It's true, I've never been into drugs. And although I won't be having Bristol Cream on Christmas morning either, I'd take an ice-cold Spanish sherry with padrón peppers over a spliff any day.

'What I'm trying to tell you, Jessica, is you find happiness through the people you choose and the people you love. You've got to find your people.'

So I tell her that when I first arrived today I was confused because, despite telling me she had no maternal longings, her house felt like a family home.

'But it feels like a truthful one to me,' she says. 'We're not forced to be family. It's a family we've chosen.'

The doorbell rings. Kim jumps up to go and answer it. It's another member of the family who has forgotten his keys.

———————

Later, in my gym pool, I swim for two hours – back and forth, back and forth – and think about the word Kim's given me for the Channel. She says it will feel great if I recite it when I'm swimming. She says it might even make me feel as spacey as a spliff. So I try it out, attempting to say the word as I'm gliding under the water. 'Om.' Ommm. Ommmmmmmmm. And for the rest of my swim, I feel like I'm in the moment and the moment's in me.

The Right Way Round

When, like Kim, I think of what my first memory is, I am about two. I'm standing in my parents' bedroom, hands on hips, looking up at their open cupboards and saying: 'Right, we've got to get these organised.' The thing about childhood memories is they get printed in your head like a photograph. I can't really have been only two years old or said those words exactly, but that's my memory. A toddler, barking orders as if I was the parent.

I can't remember whether my dad was there or whether he was at work. From before I was born he'd had a job as a finance clerk for a trade union which had its head office not far from our house in north London and he worked there until he retired. But if he was at home he'd have been sitting at the desk in their bedroom reading poetry or doing the easy crossword in the newspaper. My dad never attempted the hard crossword; he knew his limits. My mum was probably in the kitchen, cooking or standing at the counter eating; she always seemed to eat standing up. She was never a natural in the kitchen – things would take a long time and there would be a lot of mess – but she always seemed to be in there doing something. If she wasn't in the kitchen she'd be in the sitting room reading the Bible. Neither of my parents ever read novels. My dad read poetry and my mum read the Bible. As a child, I thought that, of the two, poetry was probably better.

I spent a lot of my childhood trying to coax and sometimes coerce my parents into being how I thought parents should be. I would quietly observe how my friends' mums and dads behaved and bring those lessons home. Some of these ideas were unfounded, like my childhood belief that white sliced bread was better than brown. But others still seem important – like changing the bedcovers regularly or not encouraging me to skip school so I could go shopping in town with mum instead. There were also things I hated that I couldn't change, like the fact we never had a car, which made us very reliant on other people's favours. My dad did start learning to drive before I was born but he failed his test first time and was so demoralised by the failure that he never tried again. My mum probably wouldn't have been safe behind the wheel, so it's just as well she never drove. I always say that if you looked inside her head, what you'd find is white noise, which isn't the best condition for driving. I couldn't do anything about the car so I focused on things like cupboards – tidying cupboards was something I could get done.

My dad was this strange combination of being a depressive whilst also having a tremendous *joie de vivre*. If you asked him what he thought of the world he'd say it was a terrible place. He was always full of regrets for the things he'd never done. But he loved a party, he'd always be the first to get up to dance and sing. And he'd spend hours giving me and my friends piggybacks round Boudicca's grave on Hampstead Heath. The ancient barrow (probably not actually the Celtic queen's burial mound) made a perfect circuit to work up an appetite – like me, my dad loved food. I remember the time we went on holiday to the island of Jersey. We were on the ferry and the sea was rough. Lots of passengers were being sick. Luckily I wasn't (which in retrospect may be why I thought I'd be fine on our Channel relay). Then my dad disappeared and I thought he must be ill too, until I found him in the ship's canteen with a plate piled high with all sorts of food. When I asked him how he got it – on account of the fact the canteen had closed until the sea calmed down – he told me it was amazing what people left behind on their plates. I chuckle thinking about it now, but at the time I had to reprimand him because, although he loved food, and a bargain, it wasn't really the done thing.

Unlike my dad, my mum was never a depressive, but she struggled to enjoy the pleasures of life. If you asked her whether she wanted something to eat or drink her immediate reaction would always be to say 'no'. If we ever went out to a restaurant – which wasn't often because my dad didn't like spending money – she'd choose to sit and watch us eat whilst she just had a cup of coffee. I felt I had to tell her this wasn't the done thing in restaurants either but she didn't stop doing it; she always denied herself. Maybe that's why she ate standing up, as if she didn't really deserve to sit down. Either that or she thought someone might take it away so she had to be ready to run.

Another imprinted memory I have – and this one is from when I was about seven – is losing my mum when we were at Brent Cross Shopping Centre. Looking back, I wonder whether I engineered this to test what she would do. I'd heard announcements for lost children when we'd been shopping before and I think I partly wanted to hear my name over the tannoy. I found the place where lost children go and told the lady behind the desk that I'd mislaid my mum. They did a tannoy announcement. I heard my name. They did another. I heard it again. But no one came.

The lady at the desk looked sorry for me, a child no one wanted, and I regretted getting myself lost because I knew it wasn't true. It was just that my mum probably didn't know there was a place to go for lost children and she probably didn't hear the tannoy because of the white noise. Eventually, after over an hour, the lady asked me whether I knew my home telephone number. I gave it to her and my mum answered. When she passed me the phone, mum sounded relieved I'd been found and suggested I come home on the bus. I know I should have probably saved her the trip there and back, especially as we didn't have a car, but I thought that, given she'd left me at the shopping centre and I was only seven, really it was right she came back and got me. Whilst I was waiting I wanted to tell the lady at the desk that my mum did love me, it's just she wasn't always sure what to do. Next time she'd know where to go, maybe even listen out for the tannoy, but I didn't risk testing her again.

I never blamed my parents for the way they were, I just wished it could have been different. I knew from an early age that neither of them had anyone to learn from when they were children and that's what made life hard. My mother was an illegitimate baby, born out of wedlock at a time when that status was shunned. She only met her father once, when she was a tiny girl; she says she remembers it, but I don't think she really does. He was shot and killed during the Second World War. Whether she would have met him again if he hadn't died is impossible to know.

My father also didn't really know his father and has only one memory of him and that is of them going together to the Lord Mayor's Show. I believe this memory because my dad describes it so vividly. The only other memory he has of his father is of a policeman coming to their house on Christmas Day to inform them that he had been found drowned in a stream in the Lake District. What my grandfather was doing in the Lake District on Christmas Day when his family were at home in London is not this story but it is an intriguing one.

Although neither of my parents really knew their fathers, both did have deep bonds with their mothers, though these were far from straightforward. As a single woman with an illegitimate baby, my maternal grandmother struggled to survive and consequently, my mum spent most of her early years in a children's home. My father's mother committed suicide knowing that my dad would be the one to find her, leaving him just her body on a rope with a beautiful poem beside it as a note. So you can't really blame them for not always knowing how to be parents, and although I craved rules and order, there wasn't any shortage of love.

Kim never liked her parents, and that's one of the reasons she may never have wanted to be a parent herself. I love my mum and dad. But as their child I always felt that part of my role was to teach them how to be parents and I guess, since then, I've always wanted to have a go at doing it the right way round.

The Peter Pan Cup

I nearly didn't go. I hate Christmas parties. In fact, I'm pretty much a party-hater full stop. I'm hopeless at small talk; the moment I get chatting to someone I panic about getting stuck and running out of conversation. And despite my love of food and drink there is nothing about warm alcohol and buffets that appeals. Buffets are dangerous – I always eat too much and then scold myself afterwards for spending more time at the buffet table than doing what you're supposed to do at parties, which is enjoy other people's company.

It was the Saturday morning before Christmas, the day of the Serpentine Swimming Club's annual seasonal festivities, and I was down at the lake for my weekly dip in the cold. Everyone was getting excited about the evening ahead and several people asked whether I was going. I'd bought a ticket weeks ago to show willing, but had already decided I wasn't. Things were bad at home, and I couldn't face putting on my Christmas party armour. But then someone mentioned in passing that they were looking forward to the show and my ears went into alert. The show? What show? It was only then I learned that a major feature of the annual party is the entertainment, in which various members of the club get up and perform a turn. *The Serpentine's Got Talent* was the sort of party I could manage. I changed my mind and said yes.

The location was a village hall in Barnes, south-west London, and it was like arriving at the reception of a rural wedding. A stage at one end, wooden beams and, on either side, long trestle tables laden with food. Nick and his wife were responsible for organising it all and everything was plentiful. There was the meat table, the cheese table, the sweet table and the drinks table, each manned by a different member of the club. Village-fete style, there were various games – like 'guess the bum', with photos of the posteriors of club members in their swimming costumes pinned to the wall.

And then the entertainment started, with each act getting a strict three-minute slot, which was rarely adhered to but no one cared. The plentiful line-up included a rendition of 'Swimming [as opposed to singing] in the Rain', a hilarious 'Dance of the Sugar Plum Fairy' performed by four people dressed in fat suits as if naked but for their swimming trunks, and, towards the end, an absolutely inspired version of David Bowie's 'Space Oddity' retitled 'Serpentine Oddity', with the opening line 'Changing room to Swimmer Tom . . .'

Boris was sitting behind me, and for a man who usually has the steeliest demeanour he was in raptures; he kept leaning towards me, laughing and saying, 'What do you think about this?' What I thought about this was it was extraordinary. I'd never experienced anything quite like it and one of the things that struck me was the total lack of hubris in every performance, just the joy of being together and celebrating their club and Christmas. The entertainment finished with everyone standing up, singing the Serpentine Club anthem, 'In the Duck Poo', set to the tune of 'Oh My Darling, Clementine', lungs raised high to the rafters. And after this, the chairs were stacked to the sides and dancing began. Young and old tangoing together in happy abandon. I guess you had to be there to understand and I'm glad I was.

Five days later, 25 December, I am at the lake again for the annual Christmas Day race. It's called the Peter Pan Cup. It's been held every year since 1864, and in the early 1900s became associated with J. M. Barrie – creator of the boy who never grew up – who presented the prize for many years. It's the most prestigious day of the club's calendar and the banks of the Serpentine are crowded with onlookers. The excitement in the changing room is palpable. We each get given a black hat with a white number on it. This is not regular race protocol. This is Peter Pan protocol. I am number forty.

The race is due to start at 9 a.m. sharp but there is a delay. Someone who went in the water earlier has collapsed due to the cold and an ambulance has had to be called. This has created a lot of kerfuffle and has increased the suspense and anticipation amongst the swimmers and the crowd. After the ambulance has left – assurances given that the swimmer is going to be fine – everyone starts to file down to the starting line, which is along the pontoon. The crowd is cheering, the atmosphere like a Roman amphitheatre, the cold water our wild animal. We line up, hands to our chests, huddling together to keep warm. The counter starts counting, and when my handicap time comes I get in. I swim. The cold catches my breath, the thrash of bodies around me both a comfort and a curse. The noise from the crowd increases. I swim. I swim. I swim.

Did I come first? No. Did I come last? Not quite. This wasn't to be the year I would hold the Peter Pan Cup high. But the next morning on the front page of a national newspaper there I am, standing on the pontoon with my fellow Serpentine swimmers with the number forty on my hat. The headline: 'The Swimmers Who Really Earned Their Christmas Dinner'. And I think of that other newspaper I was in and that other headline and I smile.

———

The first verse of the Serpentine anthem goes:

Swim in Duck Poo – That's What We Do
Come on in – the water's fine
You are in – my heart forever
Oh my darling – Serpentineeeeeeeeeeeee

I love these people. These mad, marvellous people with their strange and certain masochistic pleasure in the cold. They are starting to feel like family.

The Iron(wo)man

'My husband died.'

This morning at the Serpentine I met the most incredible woman. Her name is Eddie Brocklesby and when she was seventy years old she became Britain's oldest Ironman, or should I say, Ironwoman. Before I started training for the Channel I didn't know what an Ironman was. If asked, I might have hazarded a guess that it was something to do with weightlifting, but I now know it's an ultimate endurance race that involves swimming for 2.4 miles, cycling for 112 miles and then running a marathon of 26.2 miles. In that order. Without a break. And generally in a strict time limit of seventeen hours, maximum. As far as I can see the only good thing about an Ironman is that the swimming bit of it is relatively short.

Eddie, who took up running in her fifties before adding in cycling and swimming, had only previously been in a housewife's netball team and done a bit of ballroom dancing. She's now seventy-two and still at it. I ask her to swim with me for inspiration and then take her for breakfast to chat. We order coffee and eggs from the Serpentine Lido café and head out to the round metal tables and chairs that line the lake. If you're lucky you can get one right by the water's edge where you can watch the swimmers and commune with the ducks. Eddie has a small, well-toned frame and a shock of curly henna-red hair, and when I acknowledge the obvious – that she doesn't look her age – she tells me it's one of the two most frequent things people say to her. The other being they wish their mother or father would do what she's doing. Forget the parents, I wish *I* could do what she's doing. But it's an extreme sport for anyone, let alone a septuagenarian, and I'm keen to know what's driving her.

She laughs. 'You want to swim the Channel and you're asking me?'

'Yeah, well, I'm looking for answers. Why go to such extremes?'

'I don't think I was aware that I was, really,' she says. 'I started by doing half-marathons in Nottingham, where we used to live. The race was in a lovely figure of eight so that you came back to Holme Pierrepont at Trent Bridge at the halfway point, and it did seem to me that all the emaciated, sad-looking people were going on to run the full marathon and all the healthy ones were stopping halfway. I remember noticing that. And then' – she pauses for a second – 'my husband died.'

She doesn't need to say any more. Those three words are enough to give me my answer. Not just for Eddie, but also for me. Nicola Horlick was right: it's grief that has driven us to these extremes. Eddie's grief is the loss of a husband of thirty years and the father of her three children; and mine is the loss of the children I never had and now, I fear, the father I was never able to introduce them to. So, I do have the answer. I am swimming my way out of grief. Water has become my drink and my drugs: when I'm training, it takes control and that feels good, and when I get out after another gruelling session, for the rest of the day, I feel that at least I've achieved something positive. Although I started this endeavour because I wanted to do something big, I've come to love the little things, like the smell of chlorine on my skin after I've been in the pool, and the pleasantly tingly sensation when I get out of the cold of the lake before the shivers of the afterdrop hit.

I ask my iron(wo)man for a word, and the one she gives me is 'opportunity'. Eddie says she wants people to know that age is an opportunity – the reverse of what people usually believe, which is that getting older means decline. But what she's made me realise this morning is that grief is an opportunity too: to do something in your life that you might never have done without it and which, in the end, might be the only thing that gets you through.

The Politician

"'Carpe diem" – make the most of what you've got.'

I guess with an address like 'Portcullis House' you should expect security. It's a good job I'm on time because my bag has to go through one of those airport-style machines before I can even reach reception. After I've given my name and received an identity badge, I take a seat in the waiting area. A few minutes later, the parliamentary secretary to the Member of Parliament for Slough comes to collect me and leads me upstairs. I think about trying out my opening line on him to see how it goes down – 'So, who did more damage, John Betjeman or David Brent?' – but before I get the chance he opens a door on the left and shows me into the office of Fiona Mactaggart MP.

We shake hands. I reach into my bag and take out my offering – a tin of flourless cakes. I'd been given the tip off that she was 'wheat free' and had got them from a health food store near to work. She thanks me but doesn't offer me one, which is a shame because I was rather looking forward to seeing how they tasted. I sometimes wonder whether I could be wheat- or gluten-intolerant myself. Such a lot of people seem to be these days, and Dr Google could probably find me a link to infertility. But then I think: *Why would I want to know? I'd have to give up bread*, and move on.

'Look at what we're debating,' she says as soon as I sit down, pointing towards a screen behind me in the corner of the room. It has the words 'Human Embryology and Fertilisation' written in white across a green background. It seems a sort of happenstance, but I'm confused as to what it means and don't know how to ask without looking stupid.

Fiona carries on talking: 'Actually, it's not about IVF in general. It's about mitochondrial transfer.'

I'm still none the wiser and do that thing that people who don't want to appear stupid do: I nod and don't ask. Instead, I enquire where the debate is happening and she tells me it's in the Chamber and she'll take me over to have a look if there's time. Does she mean the House of Commons? How would we get there? We're not actually in the Parliament building, we're over the road in a rather modern-looking office block with a lot of glass which belies its medieval name. Besides, surely you can't just drop into the seat of British democratic power *if there's time* and you fancy it? Can you? My lack of understanding of political protocol is clearly another reason I will never make PM.

The screen behind me dongs, like a single strike of Big Ben.

'What's that?' I ask.

'That happens when someone else gets up to speak,' she explains.

'I see,' I say, learning.

With all this going on, there just hasn't been an opportunity to ask the Slough question, so the bombs of Betjeman and Brent remain silent and we go straight to the subject of IVF. Fiona tells me she went through six rounds of treatment before giving up after she got a diagnosis of multiple sclerosis: 'I thought, "OK, I give in,"' she says. 'But at the same time I thought: "You've got to do something, dear – if you can't have children you might as well try and change the world instead. Be an MP." So I did that. It was my equivalent of swimming the Channel.'

I'm not sure what comes into my head first when she says this. Is it the realisation that here is the only woman I've met so far who, like me, has been to extreme lengths to become a mother which haven't worked? Six rounds of IVF is a lot, and getting a diagnosis of MS is a terrible trump card – or as Fiona says sarcastically, 'just joy'. Or is it that she seems to share my feeling that, if we can't become mothers, we're going to have to do something big instead?

'How old were you when you gave up?' I ask.

'About forty-three.'

That figures.

'And have you been able to change the world?

She thinks for a moment. 'Well, when I was a backbencher, I persuaded the Home Secretary to change the law in relation to British overseas citizens,' she says and then relays how people in former British colonies had the status of being British citizens, but if they were kicked out of the colony for any reason – as Idi Amin did to people of Asian descent in Uganda – they weren't allowed to come to the

UK. 'So they had a status which wasn't a nationality and I don't think countries can do that to people,' she says. 'It was the first thing that Hitler did to the Jews – take away their citizenship. And it's just wrong.' She tells me that all the civil servants said it would be a disaster if we changed the law, as a quarter of million people would flood into Britain, and that she swore to the Home Secretary that the civil servants were wrong, it wouldn't happen. He listened to her and passed the law. Fiona finishes with a flourish: 'And I was right, and they were wrong. So I changed that and righted a profound injustice.'

So here is a woman who decided to use her grief to make the world a better place for others. But the question remains: is it enough? I want to ask her more about why she went through so much IVF. She clearly loves children. She was a primary school teacher before she was a politician and has several godchildren and says she wishes she had more. She also confesses that her default reading is children's novels. She tells me she chose not to talk about her own pursuit of motherhood in public because she didn't want to disclose details about her relationship. (This immediately makes me think of what I have disclosed and what that might have done to my own relationship.) She says she only broke her rule and spoke about it once: when there was a debate in the Commons about embryo research (which a lot of people were deeply opposed to) and she wanted to speak up about the fact that she had two embryos in a freezer somewhere and objected to the fact that they could be used for research into infertility – which as a woman in her fifties was irrelevant to her – but couldn't be used for research into MS, which did affect her life. And then, as if she can read my thoughts, she suddenly says: 'Look, I profoundly regret that I'm not a parent and I feel sad about it, but actually I love my life, so you can feel both things at the same time. I suppose what I would say to women who are anxious about childlessness, is this: "Carpe diem" – make the most of what you've got.'

The screen dongs again.

'Now listen,' she says, changing the subject. 'At some point a bell is going to ring, and at that point I have to go and vote. When it rings, don't panic. I've got eight minutes.'

'OK,' I say, panicking because I haven't got anywhere near through all my questions. 'So will I leave, or do I come with you, or do I wait here?' I say, flustered.

'You can't come with me during a vote, but if we finish before this debate ends I'll take you across.'

I suggest I'd better jump to my final question and she agrees and says that if there's time afterwards we can walk and talk. I ask her for a word, explaining that I'm collecting them to motivate me to keep swimming. There's a long pause.

'You see, when you started saying that I thought: what do I do when I need motivation? And what I do is I recite to myself the poem "Ozymandias".' She begins to say it aloud and when she reaches the end, she pauses: 'That poem gets me through all sorts of things. Just the vision of that statue in the sand, who was there and was mighty and who's now crumbled to nothing and isn't. And I don't know why it enables me to do these things but I find it very supportive when my stomach muscles are about to let me down. So I'm going to give you Shelley's "Ozymandias". That's my word.'

I decide not to mention Mary Wollstonecraft or Harriet Westbrook or Mary Shelley, or how this family seems to be following me around. I just say, 'Thank you, it's a beautiful word,' because it is.

'Now come on, let's go, the debate's nearly over,' she says, getting up and leading me out into the corridor.

'How do we get there?' I ask. 'Is there a secret tunnel?'

'Something like that,' she smiles.

She starts walking briskly and I trot a few steps behind her as she leads the way along a cloistered path that links Portcullis House to the Houses of Parliament under Westminster Bridge. The place is thronging with people walking back and forth, many of whom greet us as we stride past. Then Fiona opens a door on our left and ushers me through. 'Let's go this way,' she says conspiratorially, 'we're not supposed to but it's quicker.' We head up some back stairs and emerge into a lobby area where there's a man dressed in tails. She tells me to hand over my mobile phone and bag to him. There is an urgency to her instructions, which is all rather thrilling, and I still don't fully comprehend where we are or what we're doing. As I'm waiting for the man to give me a disc with a number on it so I can retrieve my things later, a bell starts ringing furiously and Fiona says hurriedly: 'That's it, the debate's finished, I'm going to have to go and vote. We'll have to say goodbye.'

I throw my arms around her in a hasty and unwieldy hug and then she's gone.

'So what do I do now?' I ask, turning to the tailed man.

'You can go in and look if you like,' he says, pointing to an open door ahead of me. I walk through, not sure what I'm going to find, but the dark wood and green leather of the room below is unmistakable. I am in the public gallery of the House of Commons. There is a Perspex screen that separates visitors from the MPs but the space is so intimate that you still feel like you can almost touch them. I sit down, taking in everything around me in wonder. The MPs below are milling about and I'm surrounded by a large group of women. I lean over to one of them and whisper, 'What's happening?'

'They're voting,' she says.

'What on?'

'Mitochondrial transfer in IVF.'

It's the same phrase that Fiona mentioned earlier.

'What's that?' I ask, feeling braver at showing my ignorance to a stranger. The woman clearly doesn't want to engage in conversation, she seems distracted, but I press on. 'I know a lot about IVF,' I say, trying to get her to take me seriously.

'It's not about fertility,' she says with disdain. 'It's about genetic diseases.'

'Right,' I say, still confused, and then try another tack. 'I've just been with an MP who has gone to vote.'

A woman in front of me turns round and snaps: 'What way are they voting?'

'Err, I'm not sure. Yes, I think.' I hope this is the right answer.

'Good,' she says matter-of-factly and turns back to the front.

It's clear that everyone around me is very on edge. I don't dare ask another question. Then a man sits down next to me and I decide to try him instead. I lean over and whisper quietly: 'Can you explain to me what mitochondrial transfer is, please?'

He proves more amenable than the women and explains it's when a piece of DNA is removed from an embryo and replaced with someone else's, which is a way of enabling women who have severe genetic disorders to prevent passing them on to their children. It's currently banned in the UK.

'Because it technically means creating babies with three parents?' I ask.

'That's right,' he nods. 'Some say it's the slippery slope to designer babies.'

'And what's your involvement?'

'I head up the team that pioneered the research,' he says.

'Oh wow,' I reply, but before I can say anything else it seems as if something's about to happen. The Speaker of the House stands up from his throne and calls for order. The tellers stand in front of him, take a step forward and bow their heads. Then one of them holds up a piece of paper and reads: 'The ayes to the right 382. The noes to the left 128.'

A massive cheer rises up from the gallery. The women around me start to whoop and to weep, and the man standing next to me calmly smiles at the triumph of science and democracy.

The next day, reports confirm that Fiona Mactaggart was one of the 382 MPs who voted yes – so there she goes, changing the world again. This time for mothers, even though she'll never be one herself.

'Ozymandias'

I met a traveller from an antique land,
Who said – 'Two vast and trunkless legs of stone
Stand in the desert . . . Near them, on the sand,
Half sunk a shattered visage lies, whose frown,
And wrinkled lip, and sneer of cold command,
Tell that its sculptor well those passions read
Which yet survive, stamped on these lifeless things,
The hand that mocked them, and the heart that fed;
And on the pedestal, these words appear:
My name is Ozymandias, King of Kings:
Look on my works, ye Mighty, and despair!
Nothing beside remains. Round the decay
Of that colossal Wreck, boundless and bare,
The lone and level sands stretch far away.'

Percy Bysshe Shelley

When I read these words, I think not just of kings but also
of mothers. I suppose in the end everything in this world is
transitory. Not just power and success but also motherhood.
Nothing beside remains.

The Ice Queen Foster Mother

'They've all got eating problems. All of them . . .
And I was comfort eating for something missing out of my life.'

'And I got out and started feeling really cold and I thought, "I'm getting really cold now." So I ran up the stairs and I thought, "Ooh, I'm going to get in that shower." And I got in the shower and I turned on the hot tap and my body literally went a black colour. All my stretch marks went deep black and I thought, "Ooh, that's dark, Jack." So I got out of the shower and I bent down to pick my knickers up off the floor and I thought, "My heart is going to come out of my body." I thought, "Ooh, that's funny, my heart's coming out of my body." It was going bang, bang, bang. So I lay on the bed and everything was going round, and I could feel it slowing right down and I thought, "I'm going to die." I lay on the bed laughing at myself, thinking, "You're going to die, Jack, but it's not so bad, it's not so painful." And you know when they say there's a light at the end of this tunnel, well, I could see it. It was all white and this brilliant light was coming towards me but I wasn't frightened, I was euphoric.'

She stops as if remembering the moment and I don't

say a word, totally transfixed. 'And then the door opened and my husband come in,' she continues. 'He'd come home from work because he'd forgotten something and he'd been calling my name. I didn't hear him and he come in and I was lying on the bed more or less naked and I said: "Dave, quick, take off your clothes and cuddle me." Because I'd read somewhere that's what you did. Anyway he jumped next to me and he screamed out loud and said: "Christ, what have you done, Jack? You're just like a bit of pork out the freezer . . ."'

What she'd done was gone and got into the little swimming pool in their back garden in the middle of winter when it was about two degrees in temperature. What she'd done was swum for forty minutes until she thought she probably ought to get out and have a bit of breakfast. What she'd done was gone and got hypothermia, which is not a condition that is the preserve of old ladies wrapped in foil blankets, as she thought, but contractible by anyone whose body temperature drops below thirty-five degrees. It's one of the hazards of cold-water swimming. Get it bad and it can kill you; and the thing that swimmers have to be most wary of is that when you're swimming and you stop feeling the cold and start feeling euphoric, that's the time you really have to worry.

But that was then – that was before Jackie Cobell became a record-breaking Channel swimmer.

We meet for the first time for lunch at a lovely country pub near her home in Sevenoaks, Kent. She looks more glamorous than I imagined: white blonde hair, face made up, and wearing a beautiful bright pink jumper which she tells me instantly was £4.99 from Asda. Within minutes I know I could to listen to her for hours. She's a natural raconteur with the wonderful quality of being exactly who she is without any guile.

An East End girl who has always loved the sea, Jackie grew up in a tiny two-bedroom flat on a council estate, where she shared a room with her three siblings and a single bed with her brother. She tells me that whenever she got in the sea it felt wonderful to have somewhere all to herself. She wasn't a great swimmer but she loved the water – and then she grew up, got married and had a family. It took a long time for the sea to refigure in her life, but eventually it did – in a big way.

'Now I want you to have whatever you like,' I say, opening the menu. 'Because this is my treat and I'm going to.'

'I can't eat too much,' she says. 'I had a gastric bypass five years ago.'

'It's no good having a gastric bypass if you're a Channel swimmer,' I say. 'Eating is the only good thing about it.'

We both look up from the menu and smile simultaneously.

'What food do you like, then?' I ask.

'Oh, anything really. I love meat, although I don't eat a lot of it in this day and age. I find it hard to digest.'

'I loved that little thing you sent me yesterday,' I say. 'What was that animal? Was it a chicken?'

'Yeah, summat like that,' she says, laughing.

I'm referring to the Facebook confirmation of our lunch meeting. Jackie had sent me an emoji that looked like a chicken eating a burger and chips and a slice of pizza with the words 'let's eat' to the right of its feathered head. It had made me smile, even though I would never eat a burger, chips and pizza at the same time (too many carbohydrates on one plate even for me), and I knew then that it was going to be a fun lunch. Jackie tells me she's useless on the computer except for Facebook. She's always on that, though, she says, and then adds, 'bloody thing'.

I decide I might have a burger and chips (minus the pizza) and notice it comes with a slice of bacon in batter. Generally I feel the same about burgers and bacon as I do about chips and pizza – they shouldn't be part of the same dish (it's a beef-and-pork-together thing). But I don't want to look picky in front of Jackie and I have to admit that there's something about the 'in batter' that makes the bacon seem more attractive, so I decide to go with the dish as billed. Whilst I'm thinking all this, Jackie is still deciding, and eventually, as if she's been going through food conversations in her head too, she says: 'Yeah, I think I'll have the harissa-marinated beef fillet skewer.'

After we've ordered I ask Jackie to tell me where her dream to swim the Channel began.

'Well, years back, really,' she starts. 'I'd heard about this Channel thing when I was quite young but I thought it was just for athletes and stuff. And then I found out anybody could do it so I thought, right. I'd spent all my life being fat and trying to lose weight and thinking I love water and swimming but, you know what it's like, you feel self-conscious. And then I got to fifty and I thought sod 'em all. I'm going to give myself a goal in life and start training to swim the Channel. Anyway, I told my family, and my husband was all for it, but my dad said: "You'll never swim the Channel, not until Nelson gets his eye back."'

The way she says it makes us smile even though we can both see the sadness.

Following this, she tells me her dad said something like: 'You're too old and fat anyway. I bet you a thousand pounds you don't.' And then he turned round and slapped the back pocket of his trousers as if to say his money was safe. And she thought: 'Right, I'm going to show you.'

It took her six years, but she did. As it turned out she had to show lots of other people as well: when she was training in Dover everyone used to take the mickey out of her as she'd always be the first in and the last out of the water because she was so slow. But in July 2010, she set out from Shakespeare Beach (or 'Shakey,' as she calls it) one Sunday morning.

'I knew I was taking my time,' she tells me.

'Were they asking you on the boat how you were?'

'Yeah, but I didn't speak much. They ask all sorts of personal questions to make sure you're OK. I remember at one point them asking, what's your pilot's name, and I said: "It's Pilot Lance, and we're going to France, OK?"'

I enjoy the thought of Jackie popping her head out of the cold water and shouting out this rhyme in her broad cockney accent.

'One time it really roughed up,' she says. 'Then a wave caught my shoulder and twisted it right round and I felt this gristly noise. It was so painful and I thought, I don't know if I can go on, but after a while the pain, well it just becomes a feeling. It's like some person having a thousand lashes or something, it doesn't register any more.'

I listen, awestruck: 'So what was the point you knew you were going to do it, Jackie?'

'Well, I was aware it was getting dark and before I knew it the sun was coming up again. It was just like a fleeting moment and I was thinking: was that the night or a cloud over the sun? And then I looked up and saw a couple of buildings and thought, yeah, yeah, I can only be half an hour away, and then I looked up again and they were gone. I thought it was a mirage or a dream. And I remember feeling really tired. This terrible tiredness I'd never felt before but then suddenly, I felt the water becoming warmer. And they were all shouting on the boat, "Go for it, Jack, go for it." Then the water went so warm, like a bath, and they were shouting, "Put your feet down, Jack, put your feet down." And then I could feel the sand under me and I thought, "This is it, I've actually made it."'

She'd made it all right – in twenty-eight hours and forty-four minutes, making her the world record holder for the slowest Channel swim ever. And as she describes the moment she landed and then came back to Dover harbour to a welcome party of family, friends and other swimmers with flowers, balloons and cheers, I can feel the emotion of it in her and I can't hold back my tears.

'And what did your dad say, Jackie?'

'He gave me the money straight away.'

She laughs, I cry.

Since then Jackie's life has changed completely. When she got home she collapsed into bed with all her clothes on – 'all mucky and 'orrible', she says – and her plan was to stay there for a week, she was so tired. But the next morning she was woken up by her husband shaking her and saying 'the news' was coming round. Overnight her swim had made headlines around the world – 'I even had a publicist', she says proudly. On one of the television programmes she appeared on, the presenter asked her what other swims she would like to do and she mentioned Alcatraz because she'd seen the film. The next day she had a call from America asking her to come over to swim it as their guest – 'They paid for everything', she says incredulously. She's subsequently been invited round the world, and what she's realised is that, although she can't do fast, she can do cold; she's even swum the Bering Strait from Russia to America in temperatures of zero degrees. She's become known across the world as the 'Ice Queen'. Not bad going for a woman who almost died from hypothermia.

When I ask, Jackie tells me her top tips for swimming the Channel are: don't listen to other people, and do what you want to do. Perfect advice for someone (me) who has written their own training manual. And then I ask her for a word, and she laughs, as if it's obvious, and gives me 'determination'.

'I'm scared', I confess suddenly.

'What are you scared about?' she says.

'I'm scared of . . .' I stop, not knowing how to answer. 'What am I scared about?' I say aloud.

'You're scared about failing', Jackie says. 'What other people are going to think if you do.'

She's right. I'm scared about failing. Again.

Jackie leans across the table and looks me straight in the eyes and says: 'You've got to tell 'em: don't take me out unless I get hypothermia or hit by a tanker.'

And then we order pudding.

―――――――

She had a scoop of date and walnut and a scoop of pistachio. I had the same. We'd already been talking for two hours and there was still something I hadn't yet asked her. Jackie may be Channel-swimming royalty but she's also a mother and a foster mother. For twenty-three years she's been taking children into her home.

'Some stayed for a few hours, a day or a week. Some stayed for seven or eight years,' she says.

'Did you get very attached to them?'

'I was particularly attached to this one lad who had severe autism. He just loved being in water. He loved being in the bath. He loved being in the swimming pool. He loved being by the seaside. You couldn't get him out. He loved it so much, he'd get off the bus and start stripping off straight away because he didn't know the social side of being covered up. Unfortunately, he went to a home in the end because he was becoming a young man and I had to think about my kids.'

Do you think you loved him because of the swimming?

'Yeah, that's right,' she smiles, remembering him. 'He was very attached to me and my left arm. Whenever I sat down and watched the telly, he'd sit on the floor and tap my arm for hours and hours. I couldn't take it away and I was getting tennis elbow.'

My heart goes out to the boy but also to Jackie, because even if it wasn't forever, for a while they were each other's joy.

'But obviously some of them were very, very challenging,' she continues, 'and you breathed a sigh of a relief when they went.' She tells me some of the horror stories: of drugs, self-harm, stealing, violence. She says that girls are harder than boys to foster. Boys can be bad but at least you get what you see. With girls you don't know what they're up to and they're far more vulnerable to being taken advantage of. Jackie says she tells the social workers she should lock them up and take away their shoes but the social workers say she can't, it's imprisonment. Surely the best possible thing that could happen to these children is to be imprisoned by Jackie's laughter and her love. But she says things have changed and fostering is no longer simply about offering a family to a child; there are so many rules, compulsory training and ticking of boxes. Stuff, she says, like you can't have a dog bowl in the kitchen and are supposed to put a clean tea towel out every two hours (I haven't changed mine for weeks).

'What do you think fostering has fulfilled in you, then?' I ask.

'That's a very difficult question. I suppose at the heart of it you have to be of a caring nature. But I've always liked chaos in my house. I don't know why, but I like it.'

I think about our quiet house and wonder what I want and like.

Earlier, when I asked Jackie why the world became captivated by her Channel story, she said she's thinks it's because she's an ordinary person. But to me, over the course of our lunch, she has shown herself to be an extraordinary person. A woman who was never a champion swimmer until she spent more time crossing the English Channel than anyone had ever done before. A woman who has not only been a mother to her own children but to over a hundred others. And a woman who at one point in her life was twenty-three stone and had to have her jaws wired up and then a gastric bypass to lose weight.

I know I joke about my love of eating versus my desire to be just under ten stone, but, like many women – and seemingly most of the women I have met so far – I too have a complex relationship with food. Whenever I meet someone who has lost weight, my immediate thoughts are: 1) you look great, and 2) I'm jealous. They don't even need to look particularly great. Thin always makes me feel jealous. But then I reckon there aren't many women in the Western world who don't understand the competing adversaries of fasting and feasting.

I say Western world because I'm conscious that there are some countries where getting enough to eat is still a priority in itself. In Indonesia, where I spent my gap year between school and university teaching English, people would congratulate someone they hadn't seen for a while for putting on weight because it meant that they were doing well and obviously had enough money to eat. But here, the words 'you've put on weight' would rarely be paired with the word 'congratulations'. Unless of course you're pregnant. During my thirties, I definitely put on weight, and sadly never because I was pregnant. I'd like to blame all the fertility drugs but I know I was probably also comfort eating to make up for the pain I was in. There were even a couple of occasions when people mistook the expanding rubber ring round my stomach for a growing baby. And then there must have been all the occasions when people were too discreet to comment. So I am fascinated, along with everything else, by Jackie's relationship with food.

'It's quite extreme having a gastric bypass and your jaws wired up,' I say boldly. 'Do you mind me asking whether it's to do with overeating or an illness you have?'

'I've always been overweight,' she replies. 'Well, no, I suppose it started back when I was fifteen.'

'What happened?'

'Oh, nothing really, just one remark. It was when I started going out with Dave. I wasn't fat. I was podgy. Well, I was well covered, and I went to meet his parents and in front of me they said to him: "She's fat, isn't she? What are you going out with her for?"'

'They said that in front of you?' I say, shocked.

'That's what it was like in them days.'

She then tells me the next time she went round, Dave's mum said she was going to try and help her lose weight and had got her some low-calorie biscuits as a meal replacement. 'So they all had roast dinner and I had this plate with two Limmits biscuits on it.'

'They didn't give you anything else?' I say, still in shock.

'No. And if you start denying yourself you start craving. You think, "Oh, I'd love that," and you gobble it down, and then you feel guilty. And I suppose that's how I've spent my life.'

'What did Dave say?'

'He said I love you no matter what weight you are, but I didn't take that on board; you start thinking you're pretty worthless because you don't look like Twiggy. And in those days you didn't answer the adults back so I just got on with it and ate me Limmits nicely and didn't lose any weight. I've spent my whole life starving and eating and that's what I've found with fostering young ladies. They've all got eating problems. All of them, every single one of them.'

'Because of emotional problems?'

'Yeah, comfort eating. And I was comfort eating for something missing out of my life. I know what it is but I find it hard to talk about . . .'

I look across the table, wondering what it could possibly be and whether she will feel able to tell me, and then as I'm thinking this she says, 'You see, I lost my firstborn. It was like forty years ago now. And I never went to his funeral and that's really bugged me all this time. They do it all differently these days. If you lose a child, you grieve a child. They give you the child to love and say your goodbyes and that didn't happen to me.'

'He was stillborn?' I ask quietly, not wanting to interrupt.

'No, he wasn't stillborn. He was alive. I was so excited. But it was a difficult birth and afterwards I went to sleep and they put him in the nursery, or so they said. When I woke up, I thought, where's my baby? And then the sister came in and I remember her saying, "Did you bring any sanitary towels in?" And I said, "Oh no, I didn't, sorry." And she said, 'Well, you should of, and by the way your baby's dead."'

The word stops the world for a moment.

'I discharged myself within a couple of hours because all I could hear was the babies crying. And because it was a difficult birth and my feet were up in stirrups for a very long time, my sciatic nerve got caught and I couldn't walk, so I didn't go to my son's funeral. But I should have gone even if they took me in a wheelchair. It's haunted me ever since, not saying goodbye to him, and every funeral I go to brings it back. I think: "I'm going to your funeral, and I didn't go to . . ."' She breaks off and then says, 'I feel so guilty. He's buried in Watford. My husband made a beautiful wrought-iron cross. I should go there, perhaps I should . . .'

'You should,' I say, remembering my conversation with the Very Reverend Lorna Hood and her work in Scotland and wishing that somehow I could ask her to do a second funeral just for Jackie.

'It's been so long now, I'm frightened that the cross isn't there.'

'But he's there,' I say softly. 'Even if the cross isn't, he's there.'

———

That afternoon, after I get back to London, I do three hours in the pool, halfway to the magic number six. As I swim I think of Jackie and of all the women who have lost a life within them and were just expected to get on with it, without a second thought.

The Parakeet

It wasn't me who heard the squawking. In spring there's always a cacophony of birds outside the top-floor windows of our flat, it becomes background noise. But there he was: huddled in the corner of a dusty disused cupboard on the landing. A little green ball of feathered fluff. He must have dropped down from the eaves where the parakeets are nesting. He was squawking for his mother.

We didn't know what to do with him, so we left him there. We opened the cupboard door and the window next to it, hoping his parents would come and rescue him. It was Sunday afternoon. I went off for training in the pool. Four hours, working slowly upwards to my target. When I got back he had been moved into a Tupperware box lined with kitchen paper under the ladder at the bottom of the stairs. I didn't look. I couldn't. But I hoped he was OK and not too scared.

We thought he'd be dead by the morning but he wasn't, and the box came inside. I heard cooing noises from the other room and then the words, 'Well done, little fella.' It was my idea about the sesame seeds and it had worked.

He'd eaten them mixed with a mushed-up raspberry from a spoon. The RSPB couldn't offer any help, apparently, because parakeets are not indigenous birds. Every few hours he'd squawk so we'd feed him again. More sesame and raspberry, and then some cooked brown rice because that's what the internet had suggested. I didn't do the feeding. I'd lie, watching, touched by the special relationship that had developed between them.

———————

I've always loved the story of the London parakeets. Legend has it that they came from the film set of *The African Queen*, the 1950s movie starring Humphrey Bogart and Katharine Hepburn, which was partly shot at Isleworth Studios. Apparently the parakeets had been brought over for the shoot and a couple escaped and started to breed, and that's how London became the unlikely home of flocks of tropical green birds, beautiful to behold in a city where the majority of feathers are black, grey and brown.

In the film Katharine Hepburn was cast as a middle-aged spinster, a role that she arguably inhabited in real life as well. The word 'spinster' is like 'career woman' – it doesn't have a comparable masculine opposite. In Middle English it referred to a woman who spins but later it came to denote an unmarried childless woman. I suppose you could say that 'bachelor' refers to an unmarried childless man but really they are not the same. You'd never pair spinster with the word 'eligible'. Spinster is a label of shame.

We fed our baby parakeet before we went to bed. He was quiet during the night and I hoped he was sleeping. The following morning, I laid in the same position as I had the day before to watch him being fed but it was immediately clear that his heart wasn't in it. He attempted a few mouthfuls but then buried his head in the corner of the box. We opened the windows wide to let him hear the other birds, hoping it would encourage him that his world was waiting. Fifteen minutes later we tried some food again. He did his best but then moved under the kitchen roll as if hiding himself from view. His heart was heaving.

By now I was late for work. I hastily had a shower and then went into the kitchen to make some breakfast. It was chaos. Kitchen roll, raspberries, sesame seeds, brown rice, everywhere. I was angry at the mess and stormed out of the house. 'It's a bird, not a baby,' I shouted.

An hour later I called to see how he was and he had died. 'Did you kill him?' I demanded. 'Did you kill him because I shouted about the mess?' As soon as I said it, I regretted it. It hadn't been me who had taken him out of the cupboard. It hadn't been me who had rung the RSPB. It hadn't been me who had fed him from a spoon or said, 'Well done, little fella' when he ate. It wouldn't be me who buried him. But I had started to love him and for a few hours he had allowed me to love us again. I knew my accusation had ruined it.

Sometimes I think the hardest thing about what I've been through – what we've been through – is that it makes it difficult to love because you're so frightened of happiness being taken away. Today, when we lost our baby parakeet, it felt like our love and happiness had been taken away yet again.

Anonymous

'You are entitled to love a child.'

The word she gave me was *'Arigatou-gozaimasu'.* She asked if she could be anonymous. Not for her sake, but for her son's. Her own mother had been a famous religious preacher who had used her and her brother as source material for sermons. They had both hated it and she didn't want to do the same to her child without knowing how he might feel in the future.

'How old is your son now?' I ask.

'Six.'

'And how old are you?'

'Sixty-two. I've got a free pass,' she whispers, and then laughs.

I do a quick subtraction in my head. This means she gave birth aged fifty-six. I ask her how she feels about that.

'Well, a bit embarrassed, I must say, because obviously it's not normal.'

'Whatever normal is,' I interject quickly.

'Sometimes when I'm with my son people say, "Ooh, is he your grandchild . . .?" and I feel a bit disappointed they assume that.'

I feel disappointed for her too, remembering my conversation in Ibiza with Claudia Spahr about society's hostile views towards older women becoming mothers. Such honesty makes me feel I can confess that it is the thing that would worry me: the judgement of others, the implication that I was too old to be a mother. She admits she hasn't told a lot of people exactly how old she is because of that. So I ask her to tell me the story of why she did it. Why she decided to take the gift of an egg from a younger woman she'd never met. She begins by revealing that she was aged forty-nine when she thought: 'Oh shit, I forgot!'

The waitress comes over to take our order. We're meeting in a Japanese restaurant that my interviewee has suggested, so I encourage her to choose for the two of us. Whatever she orders I know I'm going to like, because I like her even though we've only just met. She continues with her story. She tells me that although she had tried to conceive with her partner in her thirties, they had experienced some fertility issues and hadn't pursued treatment because life and work suddenly took them off in other directions, and they later separated. At forty-nine, when it hit her that she'd forgotten, she says she went a little bit mad. And then she read a magazine article about egg donation and, although she thought it sounded like science fiction, she couldn't get it out of her head. She had several rounds of treatment that didn't work and was approaching fifty-five, the cut-off age in many clinics. She felt she had one last chance and had to try again even if it was just to ease her mind that she'd given it a final shot. The day of her pregnancy test she remembers dreading opening the email that came through to confirm the result, leaving it until the end of the day so she could do everything she needed to do before having to face what she assumed would be disappointment. I know that feeling. But as last chances sometimes find a way of doing, it did work, and now she is a mother.

'I feel like I'm blessed,' she says. 'This is a miracle. I have been really, really lucky and in that sense I feel like being an older mother, OK, it's a problem, but it's a minor problem because I've got my son, which is really just an amazing thing.'

'So what has it brought you?' I ask.

'Say it again?' she says. We are talking in hushed tones so the people sitting near us cannot hear. I'm not sure whether she hasn't heard me or whether she doesn't quite understand the question.

'Being a mother, having a son,' I say, 'what has it brought to your life that you wouldn't have had without it?'

She thinks for a long time before answering.

'Well, so many things,' she replies finally, 'but one thing is like, well, it's a really stupid thing, but it's like . . . school life.'

'School life?' I repeat the words back to her this time, not entirely understanding her answer to my question.

'Yes,' she says, and then with a childlike wonder she continues. 'I think it's really interesting, because I've never experienced it before: going to assembly, meeting other mothers, getting involved with things. Really for me it's very exotic.'

I marvel at her choice of words to describe what many might consider to be the mundanity of a mother's life.

'Before, I was thinking about art and never had a very grounded life,' she continues, 'and now I'm experiencing how a grounded life works. And that is very interesting for me.'

'As an artist or as a human being?' I ask.

'As a human being,' she replies quickly. 'I'm more into the local community and you don't need to travel too far to get excited about . . . like . . . just going to the local museum and seeing all sorts of strange people. Mothers and family people. For me, exotic people. I never experienced it before and it's all very interesting.'

I love this idea of her taking her son to their local museum not just to see the exhibits but to enjoy the experience of being with its other colourful and curious visitors, and then, as if a new response to my question suddenly strikes her, she adds: 'But at a more profound level, loving somebody. I don't need to feel ashamed, you know. You are entitled to love a child, aren't you?' She laughs and finishes her thought: 'That's brilliant, I find.'

It is impossible not to be moved by her articulation of the pleasure in the simple pursuits of being a mother and the legitimacy of loving your child. It feels so truthful, and recalling the beginning of our conversation I ask whether these things are enough to eclipse the difficulties – the embarrassment, the feeling of being 'not normal'.

'The time will come soon when my son becomes a teenager; I haven't experienced that yet. How *he* feels. I worry about it but then I have no choice, I have to survive.'

'And what will you say to him if he says, "I wish you were like my friends' mothers"?'

She thinks for a second and then replies, 'I might go to my counsellor.'

I tease her: 'So you're going to say to your son: "Hold that thought, I'll get back to you when I've seen my counsellor"?'

'But she's really good!' she exclaims.

We both burst out laughing. Then she shows me a photo of him, her son, admiring how handsome he is and saying that although she only has a sheet of A4 information on her egg donor and has never seen her face, she obviously got a good one. She obviously did. And then we talk about me, my journey to become a mother, followed by my journey to become a swimmer, and the greatest thing about it being how much I get to eat. As soon as I say this she pushes the plate of food between us towards me, encouraging me to eat more even though I've already had probably double what she has. The thing about sushi is it feels as if you've hardly eaten anything at all – which is fabulous – so five minutes later you're tempted by another bit and then another and end up eating loads. She points to something tasty looking and tells me to take it. I try to decline so she suggests we share it. As we're eating we start to talk about food: what she cooks at home and what her son likes to eat, and she tells me the sweetest story of how she had made something special for an international evening at his school and how everything she made was eaten and how proud he was, exclaiming: 'It's gone! It all went!' She says this mimicking the voice of a little man, her little boy.

'I can go on forever about this,' she says and laughs. 'It's very strange. Life is strange, I think. I didn't expect this.'

'Isn't that what's wonderful about life?' I reply. 'If you keep on trying, it will always find a way of surprising you and giving you pleasure, and that's why it's worth living, I think.'

It's only afterwards, when I am listening back to our conversation on my little tape machine, that I notice in the background the sound of a beautifully languid jazz version of Gloria Gaynor's anthem for women. And intertwined with our own voices on the tape are the words of: '*I will survive.*'

The word she gave me was '*Arigatou-gozaimasu*'. It means 'thank you very much' in Japanese and it was given to me on one of the most delicious evenings of this life I've got to live.

The Publisher

Dear Ms Hepburn
1 – No
2 – 'Courage'
3 – Peaches
Best wishes,
Diana Athill

That's the legendary publisher Diana Athill, aged ninety-seven, answering my email.

The Restaurateur

'We're all driven by selfish things. It's just that some
selfishness is good for other people and some isn't.'

'How's your peach?'

'Absolutely delicious,' she says. 'Have a bit, I'll peel you an end.'

I'm not sure how you peel an end of a peach but if anyone knows, she does. There had only been one left, otherwise I might have had one myself, but instead I've ordered a slice of carrot cake. The peach looks better; it's one of those small, slightly squashed ones with velvet red and yellow skin. She peels and cuts me a little piece and I taste it.

'Mmm, it's good,' I say, and then for some reason I feel the need to confess that I'm about to eat my second cake of the day, which is a lot, even for me. Maybe that's why I chose carrot, in the delusion that it was somehow healthier. I tell her I had a cronut for breakfast this morning. 'Have you ever had one?' I ask.

'No. What's a cronut?' she says.

Delighted to be teaching her something on a subject she knows far more about than me, I explain that it's a deep-fried cross between a croissant and a doughnut.

'Darling,' she says. 'I think this is off my diet. I am not swimming the Channel.'

'It was rather marvellous,' I tell her, and although she doesn't seem tempted she does proceed to tell me about the most-bad-for-you thing she's eaten recently, which was a slice of brioche, heavily buttered, covered in caramelised sugar, butterscotch sauce, toasted hazelnuts, fried bananas (two of them) and ginger ice cream. Now that sounds good and is definitely on *my* diet.

When I set out on this journey to find women to meet and eat with me and talk about motherhood, I knew I had to find a chef. I secretly hoped we would have lunch, maybe that whoever it was might even cook for me, but Prue Leith is a busy woman – she didn't have an available lunch slot for months – and although I wasn't anticipating that she would only eat a modest peach and I a slightly stale-looking slice of carrot cake in the Royal Academy of Arts café, it didn't matter, because we'd bonded over the brioche.

Prue Leith's name is synonymous with food. Good food. She originally carved out her reputation running a catering business and then a Michelin-starred restaurant. She subsequently founded one of the most famous cookery schools in the world, became a judge on the successful TV series *Great British Menu* (and more recently on the even more successful *Great British Bake Off*) and her books, along with Mrs Beeton's, are the ones I turn to if I need to know how to cook anything.

Prue's motherhood story is also fascinating. When I ask her to tell me more about it, she laughs. 'We'd always say: "We've got one home-made and one off the shelf."' She tells me that originally her husband didn't want to have children because he had firm views about there being too many people on the earth already. But Prue really did, so eventually they had one and then, as neither of them wanted to bring up an only child, they adopted the other.

'What worried me desperately was that I wouldn't love the adopted child as much as my son, Daniel,' she says, broaching the question I most want to ask before I've even looked for the courage to ask it. But then, instead of elaborating, she tells me the story of how a little Cambodian girl called Li-Da, orphaned during the time of the Khmer Rouge, came into their lives. By the time Prue met her, this little girl had already lost four mother figures in her life: her biological mother; an adoptive mother who suddenly died; a nanny who had looked after her for eight months after this; and another woman who was going to adopt her but then didn't because she started going through a divorce. Prue and her husband were strongly advised against taking Li-Da because she was likely to be psychologically damaged by all the upheaval. And the woman who had been planning to adopt her told Prue that she was very naughty, drank her own bathwater and hated men. But Prue says she vividly remembers her husband sitting down on a stool and putting his arms out, and Li-Da just toddling into them with a big smile on her face. 'I thought, so much for hating men. And she's been no trouble at all, she's been wonderful. I was nervous about whether I would love her as much as my son and I used to torment myself over which one I would save if we were in a sinking boat and, within a week, I knew I would save the nearest, because it wasn't an issue.'

So there's my answer.

We talk about the adoption process: how it's never straightforward, and much less so now than it was then. Prue knows a lot about it and provides me with insights that I'd never really thought about, such as how birth control decreased the supply of babies being put up for adoption and that the majority of children needing adoption now have often had a terrible start in the world, with biological parents who have severe problems themselves. This has driven many people to try to adopt from abroad. But although there are masses of children in the developing world who need new families as a result of war, famine or social prejudice, foreign governments have become increasingly and legitimately concerned about the dangers of baby-farming – people having babies for money who are at risk of being sold into abuse and slavery and horrible things. And as if these factors alone don't make things complicated enough, there is now an obsession with checking out whether people who want to adopt a child are the right kind of parents. Prue lists all the things that influence social workers' decisions, like if you smoke and if you are the right match for a child's ethnicity. 'What if a child has a Portuguese father and a Namibian mother?' Prue says defiantly. 'How are you going to easily find a match for that?' This makes me remember my conversation with Jackie Cobell, who had told me about all the social worker rules she has to follow as a foster mother including the ones about dog bowls and new tea towels every two hours.

I think about Li-Da, a tiny toddler from the killing fields of Cambodia, who ended up with two white South African parents who had made their home in England, and a father who Prue says smoked like a chimney, and I know what I think. I think far better to have parents who want you – whoever they are, however you came by them – than not have any at all.

I like Prue Leith a lot. And not just because of the peach or the brioche. I like her because she's clever and warm and honest. Maybe this is why I feel I can tell her my deepest fears about adoption. The more I think about it, the more I see that my pursuit of motherhood has been fundamentally selfish. Prue's husband is right: it's not like the world needs any more people. It's been about me and my desperate desire to become a parent. But I don't think you should go into adoption or fostering thinking like this because, in part, your role is always going to be to look after someone else's child, and if you're going to do that job well, surely you have to put the child's needs and happiness first, not your own. I therefore feel it would be a mistake to go into it without fully coming to terms first with the fact that what I really wanted in this world was a baby that I'd made with the man that I love. Because like Camila Batmanghelidjh said, it all goes wrong when we engage in emotional pretences.

'Relax,' Prue says when I tell her all this. 'We're all driven by selfish things. It's just that some selfishness is good for other people and some isn't. I really don't think you should worry about that, but what I do think you need to be really clear about, if you consider adoption, is what you think you can cope with. You've got to think: "How resilient am I?" Most adoptions don't work because the children can be so difficult to bring up, and what a child doesn't need is to end up in foster care after three years because someone's not been able to cope.'

'And does it go wrong a lot of times?' I ask.

'Yes, I think it does,' she nods. She doesn't know what the statistics are but she tells me that generally people seem to be more successfully brought up by their own biological parents. She's not sure whether this is about class, nationality, geographical area or genes but, she says, the fact is that when it's your own flesh and blood, you know that you're responsible for absolutely everything about that child, including the way it behaves, but if you've got the baby from somebody else, the instinctive thing is to blame that somebody else if it's difficult.

In the small and crowded café, I wonder whether anyone is listening in on our conversation. I lean in and lower my voice for my next question.

'Prue, there was something else I wanted to ask if you don't mind . . . I know you and your husband had an affair before you were married. My partner and I had one as well. He's also older than me and I've always had a problem with that; I know your husband was too. I worry that somehow our relationship is wrong and all that we've been through is my retribution.'

'That's got to be nonsense,' she says immediately.

'Really?' I say, hardly believing that I am daring to share this with a stranger.

'But I do suppose,' she says more slowly, thinking through what I've just said, 'in a way I have the reverse feeling – that I don't deserve the happiness I've had. Such a good marriage, such lovely kids, such a great career. I have had it very good and I do often feel if the sword of Damocles fell on me tomorrow it would be fair cop . . .'

'I'm glad you said that, because I was thinking you've had it good. Have you had any sadness at all?'

'I think I have the nature that tends to look forward not back. I mean, I never really felt guilty about falling in love and having an affair because I know I couldn't have done anything else. And I made him happy, and he made me happy . . . I suppose one thing that is sad is that I wanted more children, either adopted or natural, and I did get pregnant again when the children were about three, but I just looked at my husband's face when I told him and it was one of absolute crestfallen horror. He was old and tired and we'd just got two toddlers beyond the twos and there I was proposing to have another one. So we didn't have it, we had an abortion, and I certainly always regretted that and . . . I still to this day find myself calculating . . .' she pauses.

'Calculating?' I repeat the word back to her.

'I don't know why, but I was convinced it was a girl and I find myself thinking, well, she'd be thirty-six now.' And then Prue leans forward and pours some more tea to fill the silence.

Like it was a soundtrack for this moment, Ella Fitzgerald's

wistful 'Into Each Life Some Rain Must Fall' comes into my mind. All the women I've met over the last year are teaching me that everyone has their sadness – even Prue.

When the music in my head stops I tell her I always wanted lots of children too. That I dream of a farmhouse table laden with food and surrounded by family and that by not becoming a mother I feel like I've been denied the opportunity of ever achieving any of this as well.

'I think you've absolutely hit something bang on there. I think this is common, not just to women but to cooks. They all get their satisfaction from feeding other people and giving pleasure. People often ask me, "What's your favourite thing?" and, well, my favourite thing is to be at the end of the table doling out cassoulet or shepherd's pie to a lot of family and friends. I like this thing of being the provider and doing really delicious food and people thinking it's lovely, and all of that, so I absolutely agree, but I tell you what, I've never been a very good mother.'

'Really?'

I'm taken aback by her sudden confession.

'No. Li-Da turned out to be a hot swimmer and we used to go the local swimming baths, and one day a trainer fellow came along and said, "Your daughter's amazing" – she was, she was like a fish in the sea. He asked if she could come to his swimming classes and I knew this would lead to me – and this is very selfish – but I knew it would lead to me going to swimming galas all the time and spending my weekends sitting on a wet bench waiting for my daughter to plough up and down the bloody pool and I couldn't think of anything worse so I said no. I remember lying through my teeth and saying she does riding every week and she's very keen on that, and she didn't even like riding very much but I had to get rid of that idea, so I was never the good mother in the sense of putting the children first; I always put me first, or at least the idea of family first.'

I think that if she had been my mother she wouldn't have been in any danger of having to sit through swimming galas because I was never in any. But it also makes me wonder about the possibility of having an adopted daughter who might not be Molly but could still be my fish. Maybe we could make a pact: I didn't get what I wanted, you didn't get what you wanted, but we did get each other, and maybe that could be enough?

At the very end of my conversation with Prue, when I ask her for a word, she gives me 'doggedness'. She says it seems to her that most success in life depends on it, but also that it makes her think of doggy paddle and a determined little thing swimming across the Channel.

And then a question suddenly strikes her: 'Can you lie on your back and rest?'

It's one I've been asked many times now because people can't believe you can swim the Channel in one go.

I tell her no.

'It doesn't work?' she asks. 'You'd start drifting in the wrong direction or something?'

'You can't stop because you'd get cold and, besides, every moment you stop is just another moment you've got to swim.'

'Ah,' she says, 'I see.'

Prue Leith is right. Swimming the Channel, like life, is all about doggedness, but the question is, can this doggy keep swimming?

Camp Eton

The children's abacuses confuse me. What are they doing at the end of each lane? But there is no time to ask; people are already ploughing up and down. I'm late. I go over to Nick (Serpentine Nick), who tells me to get into the last lane: the slow lane. I admit I do feel a bit disappointed. There are a couple of ladies of a certain age from the Serpentine already in it. They are training for a Channel relay this summer and are even slower than me, and I have to keep overtaking them. I look wistfully at the swimmers in the next lane up. I'm sure I could have a go at keeping up with them but, after all my lonely hours in the pool this winter (it is now Easter weekend), I am still the underdog.

It reminds me of the word Prue gave me, but not in a good way. Yet at the same time I am happy to be here, so I don't say a thing and after about twenty minutes a man called Jeremy joins our lane. He's about the same speed as me, so we begin swimming together and I cheer up a bit.

'Here' is Eton, the English school that needs no introduction. It has educated generations of the aristocracy, no less than nineteen prime ministers, and even Prue Leith's son. Serpentine Nick is one of its maths masters and every year the school generously allows him to hold a boot camp for aspiring Channel swimmers, mainly from our club. It's called Camp Eton. It costs next to nothing and is yet another generous gesture from this incredible community I have stumbled into. I feel very privileged, and not just because of the location.

The weekend comprises a series of swim sessions interspersed by lectures. John is here. So is 'The Catch' Ray. John's giving a talk on mental preparation. Ray is talking technique. I'm looking forward to the lectures more than the swimming – I'd still rather use my head than my arms and my legs. Actually, I am most looking forward to the all-you-can-eat Chinese on Saturday night, although once sated the next thing on the agenda after bed will be the revered and feared hundred hundreds, which take place first thing on Sunday morning. This, I learn, is when the abacus comes into its own.

But before we even get to prawn crackers, the lectures are blowing my mind. I'm only a few months off my swimming slot and I realise there is still so much I've got to learn . . . about feeding, hydration, hypothermia, fatigue, pilots, support crews, equipment, tides, tankers and training . . . and then there is something else I haven't even thought of yet: the four Ps. Nick – the sort of teacher you'd never mess around – stands at the front of the classroom and asks us to shout out what we think the four Ps of the Channel could be. Someone says 'positivity'. Another suggests 'persistence'. A third person proffers 'practise' and then we all wrack our brains for a fourth until someone shouts out, laughing, 'pain?' Nick smiles wryly before telling us that the four Ps of the Channel are in fact: 'Pee, poo, puke and periods.'

After the laughter has died down – his pronouncement having sent us all into sniggering shock – Nick tells us that not being able to pee is serious and has stopped many a swim as it becomes incredibly painful. You therefore need to get your support crew to ask you regularly whether you've been, although I'm fairly confident that my bladder will not let me down as I've discovered there is nothing nicer than a pee in cold water. (When I'm in the Serpentine I've got into the habit of treating myself to one when I get to the end of a lap.) However, poo is another matter entirely. Me and the brown stuff don't get on. Whenever I'm stressed it features in my dreams in a big way: generally, I find myself in situations when I'm trying to get away from it and can't. While Nick tells us its appearance in the Channel is relatively rare (apparently the cold makes it retract), sometimes the urge does come so you've got to be prepared, especially as faeces float. Nick's sage advice is to position yourself horizontally, then gently tread water while you pull your costume aside so that the offending substance can be offloaded with the minimum of fuss and then you can quickly scull away. Ugghhh. I tell you, I'd better be retracting and not extracting.

The third 'P' – puke – is apparently another relatively common symptom of Channel swimming which I haven't yet had to endure. Although I was sick on the boat during our relay, I haven't been sick in the water. But vomiting on a solo is often caused by nerves. Nick warns us that a sick swimmer makes the guttural sound of an animal dying. (To be honest there have been times when I've sounded a bit like that and I wasn't even sick.)

And finally: periods. I never thought that swimming the Channel would give me yet another reason to dread their arrival. Ideally, you don't want to come on just as you're about to swim. Changing a tampon in the water is not an option and if you weren't to change it there would be a danger of toxic shock. Some women decide to go on the pill in advance of their swim (oh the irony) and others just get on with it and bleed. I think if it happens I'll just get on with it. Knowing my luck where periods are concerned, it will probably happen.

After a full-on first day and a delicious supper, Sunday morning dawns, and the spectre of the hundred hundreds. A word of explanation is probably necessary here. The length of the pool is twenty-five metres. Four lengths of the pool equals 100 metres. Multiply four lengths by a hundred to make a hundred hundreds. That's 400 lengths. A child's abacus generally has ten rows of ten coloured beads. Each time we swim four lengths we push a bead across. Each time we push ten beads across, we move on to a new row of colours. When all the rows are complete we've done a hundred hundreds or in other words 10k.

Even the strongest swimmers approach the task with trepidation. Everyone starts at the same time and gradually, the hours pass and from the fast lane downwards people get through their beads. The lady relayers in our lane are let off the full amount and eventually, it's just Jeremy and me left in the pool, although he has gone and muddled things up for us because at around the midway point he got out for one of the four Ps. He was away for ages (it must have been P2) and eventually, I carried on swimming as I couldn't bear to wait any longer. I got through several beads on the abacus before he got back. We then carried on swimming together, but it's meant we are now out of synch. Some of the other swimmers who have finished come to cheer us on. And then when we finally get to the end, after three-and-a-half exhausting hours, Jeremy suddenly decides to do the lengths he missed when he was in the toilet. I was really hoping he wouldn't, but as he's been my swimming companion this weekend it seems only right to keep him company, so I carry on with him for the final few hundreds, meaning that I actually swim more than anyone else that Easter morning.

To be honest, although it's typical of my rotten luck, I don't think much of it as last week I did five hours on my own in the pool (although admittedly under less pressure). But of course no one else knows about Jessica's Channel Swimming Manual, and it turns out that those extra few lengths impress everyone because no one had been expecting me to complete the hundred hundreds. And then I did. And then I even did some more.

The following weekend, I achieve six hours in the pool. I do it at the Oasis, the beautiful outdoor swimming baths (heated, admittedly) in Covent Garden. It's one of London's hidden gems, open to the public year round – all hail the politicians and civil servants who haven't closed it to save money. In fact – top tip – the indoor pool is often colder than the outdoor one so it's worth braving the dash from the changing rooms even if there's snow on the ground. At hour four, when I stop to take a drink, I notice a man in the next lane watching me. He leans over and says, 'I've never seen anyone drinking from a flask in a swimming pool before. What's in it?'

I detect a sense of superiority and scorn in his voice. I tell him it's Maxim, an energy drink, but before I can explain that I'm swimming for six hours, he scoffs, 'Have you got a sandwich with you as well?' He ducks under and swims off before I can even reply. I feel like chasing after him and saying, 'Do you know what mate, no self-respecting swimmer I know would ever wear a nose clip.' I'm fuming for a good while; at least it passes some time.

Two hours later I do it: I achieve six hours in the pool. Fifteen minutes before the end, the most special thing of all is that I look down and see two size-twelve feet that I immediately recognise. They have come to keep me company for the final few lengths. On that landmark Sunday afternoon in the Oasis, I want those feet to swim with me forever, but soon afterwards I lose hope that they will.

The Divorce Lawyer

'There are certain tremor lines in a marriage or catalysts to divorce and IVF is high on the list.'

Before I even get to the end of my spiel she says: 'Has it put a strain on your relationship?'

I'm taken aback. Maybe she thinks I'm looking for a divorce lawyer. But she is Fiona Shackleton, divorce lawyer to princes and pop stars, not to paupers. All we've got is debt. Thousands and thousands of pounds of debt from all the IVF.

When I wrote to Fiona she invited me to afternoon tea at the House of Lords – she's my second baroness of the year – and the first thing she says as she greets me in the entrance lobby is that she never agrees to meet anyone. She says 'anyone' with definition and I think the subtext of this is that generally people only want to talk to her about her famous clients: the Prince of Wales, Paul McCartney et al., and she doesn't want to talk about them. But as she leads me along the corridors to the peers' dining room – greeting everybody we pass, including the staff, who nod and say, 'Hello, m'lady' – she tells me that there was something about my email that made her think: I must meet this woman. Maybe as a mother herself she felt for what I'd been through. Maybe the eating bit intrigued her – she started her working life not as a lawyer but as a professional cook. Or maybe it was the swimming, because one of the first things she tells me is that she swam competitively as a child. In fact, it transpires that she used to swim at Swiss Cottage, the same pool that my mum and dad occasionally took me to on Sunday mornings.

Whatever it was that made Fiona agree to meet me, she has taken my request to eat very seriously. When we reach the dining room, the waiter shows us over to a table that is set for two. One of the place settings (just one) has afternoon tea laid out in front of it: a plate of sandwiches covered in cling film, presumably to keep them fresh; two scones with jam and cream; and a slice of dark sticky fruit cake. Fiona tells me that she ordered it earlier in case they ran out and then immediately quizzes the waiter as to whether he's given me the most fattening cake they've got. She explains to him that I need to eat a lot as I am training to swim the Channel. I adore her for this instantly, so when she asks me whether the IVF has put a strain on our relationship, I don't try to evade; I nod.

'There are certain tremor lines in a marriage or catalysts to divorce and IVF is high on the list,' she says.

'Is it?'

I don't know why I'm surprised, but I am.

'Oh, without a doubt.'

'If it's successful or if it isn't?' I ask.

'Normally if it's not successful. I mean all relationships are not perfect. There is no such thing. It doesn't exist. Anyone that says that is not telling the truth. Some days you love your other half better than you love them other days. But there's something about IVF, the indignity of it, the mechanical sexual relationship, the actuation of blame. It's incredibly stressful.'

She glances down at my hand.

'Aren't you married, or do you just not wear a wedding ring?' she enquires.

Again, I'm taken aback. No one has ever asked me this before.

'No, we're not married,' I say.

'Did you not want to get married?'

'Yes ... well ... maybe ... no.'

It's another question I'm not prepared for, but I recover myself and, being honest again, admit that we were both in other relationships when we got together, which resulted in a lot of pain. We still carry the guilt from this, which is probably one of the reasons why we never got married. 'But we've been together nearly fourteen years now,' I say.

'Oh my goodness, that's quite a long marriage,' she replies.

It's the first time I've ever thought of our relationship as a marriage but it's not the first time I've wondered whether things might have been different if we actually were married. Maybe the IVF would have worked because it would have looked like we really meant it.

Fiona Shackleton is weighing me up and I wonder what's she's thinking. No marriage. No kids. No money. In her world of prenuptials, mid-nuptials and high-stakes divorce, our situation is not what she's used to. Her own marriage and motherhood story is straightforward by comparison. Still married after many years to the father of her children, two girls. If I'm honest I hadn't really planned on asking her too much about that. What I wanted to know was, when relationships break down, how does having children – or not – fit in; did they make you happier, or did the anger and pain of the breakdown hurt more than the love of your child?

'Well, of course, it's always easier when they don't have children,' Fiona says, 'but then you're not bringing a third party into a dispute, so logistically it's easier.'

'And what's it like when they do have children?'

'There's no general rule. Good parents will compromise about the children because it's not their fault you're getting divorced. And responsible parents are brave enough, whatever they may feel about their spouse – and they can be very provocative and very difficult about their partners – to overcome that for the love of their children. I sometimes say to them: "I understand you are very hurt, but do you hate your spouse more than you love your child?"'

'And does anyone ever say yes?' I ask, intrigued.

She laughs. 'They don't actually say yes, they say, "That's interesting."'

We both laugh, knowing exactly what she means.

'Sometimes people ask me if I've ever been shocked,' she says. 'And the answer is probably not – except for one particular case, when before I opened my mouth to talk about the children, my client said: "We have a problem:

neither my wife nor I want them."' Fiona then proceeds to tell me the story – mentioning no names, of course. It has a happy ending because Fiona managed to persuade her client to take the children and he was ultimately pleased that he did.

She's good, Fiona. Disarmingly charming and surprisingly self-deprecating. She says she suffers from imposter's syndrome and has overshot her limitations, and there's something in the way she says it that makes me think it's not a ruse; it's how she really feels, even though it's hardly true. I can see why you'd want her to represent you, and you'd be fearful if she were on the other side. She tells me she's a very good friend and a very bad enemy. I can see that just from the way she handles me over the scones and the sandwiches.

'What are you going to have next?' she says suddenly. 'You're not doing very well. Are you going to skip the sandwiches?'

'I *am* doing well,' I say defensively. 'I've had two scones.'

She was right; I had decided to skip the sandwiches.

'Well, we'll get another scone then,' she says.

'No, no, no,' I say, attempting to be assertive. 'Don't get me another.'

'Right, will you have a bit of cake then?'

'I might have a bit of cake. In a minute,' I say, trying to placate her. But my delay tactics go unheeded and she waves over another one of the waiters.

'You really are going to make me fat,' I say.

She dismisses this in an instant with the words: 'You can swim another mile,' and then introduces me to the waiter.

'This is my friend,' she says. 'He'll get anything for us. She's got to have something else.'

'I'll bring more scones, m'lady,' the waiter suggests.

'No, don't bring any more scones,' I implore – two scones with jam and cream is enough even for me – 'I'm going to try a bit of that fruit cake,' I say, hoping to get the two of them off my plate.

I fail.

'What other cakes do you have on offer today?' Fiona asks.

'But I like fruit cake,' I say in its defence.

'She's swimming the Channel, we've got to feed her up,' Fiona says, ignoring me.

'I'm going to sink at this rate.'

'She said she wanted to eat with me to put on weight,' she explains to the waiter.

'I'll bring the cake tray, m'lady,' he says.

'Yes, why not. Bring the cake tray to see if there's anything she prefers,' Fiona says, pleased.

I look at the fruit cake and want to give it a shrug as if to say, 'What can I do?' Fiona is a woman who knows how to get her own way. When I ask her for her word, she immediately replies, 'Can it be two?' The negotiator through and through.

The two words she gives me are 'keep going', which is rather apt considering the amount she's making me eat. She, on the other hand, has not eaten a thing, and given that she has the sort of frame that wouldn't last five minutes in the Channel, I'm interested in finding out more about her relationship with food. I'm never sure I believe that someone really cares about food if they don't eat a scone when it's on offer. So I ask her about how she came to train as a Cordon Bleu chef, and she tells me this is rubbish and that she didn't. She says the internet is full of things about her that aren't true and she never bothers to correct them. I'm surprised at this from a lawyer but she says that if you correct one thing, then you have to correct everything, which I suppose is a good legal defence.

So she never trained as a Cordon Bleu chef, but she did start cooking as a child, although she didn't learn at her mother's knee as many cooks do. She says that her mother was far more interested in speaking on the telephone and watching the 3:20 at the races than spending time in the kitchen. Fiona tells me her mother was the sort of person who would leave the onions out of a beef bourguignon because she didn't like them and then wonder why it tasted terrible. So Fiona learned from a book, a French recipe book for children, and her first creation was *steak au poivre*. After that she didn't look back. Although she trained as a solicitor, her first job was catering for private dinner parties and it was at one of these she had her own *My Fair Lady* moment. As she handed out the bread rolls, the businessmen round the table were discussing the need for a solicitor to negotiate the purchase of some of their company's shares, and she couldn't stop herself from saying, 'Under Section 35 of the Companies Act 1980 you can't buy your own shares.' Well, that was the end of her cooking career. By her mid-twenties she was a partner in a law firm. Now she's the one sitting round the table at high-level dinners being handed the bread rolls, although it doesn't look like she eats many.

When I say this to her she says she hasn't always been this size. She tells me that for years she was constantly dieting, but then when she put her hourly charge rate up she experienced a seminal moment that changed everything: 'I'd skipped breakfast and the client was telling me some story and I was looking at the biscuits, and I'm thinking, shall I eat the biscuits? Shan't I eat the biscuits? Shall I eat the biscuits? Shan't I eat the biscuits? And then I thought, "This is robbery,"' – she thumps the table as she says this – 'I thought, "Fiona, you can't charge this woman £250 an hour and be worrying about whether you eat the biscuits or not." So after that I stopped dieting and always had breakfast. So when the biscuits come in, I don't even look at them, all I'm thinking about is what my client's telling me, and when I stopped dieting I was a much better size than when I was always watching what I was doing.'

I reflect on all the work meetings that I've sat through dreaming about food. There have been many of them. This is why Fiona's so good; she understands the female psyche. There are women everywhere who are enslaved to diets that will never work or who are comfort eating to numb their pain, like Jackie Cobell and the girls she fosters. The seminal moment that changed things for Fiona was putting up her hourly rate to £250 and mine was deciding to try and swim twenty-one miles. If the Channel never gives me anything else, it's given me that: a justification to eat whatever I want for a positive purpose and without feeling guilty.

The waiter comes over with the cake tray.

'We don't have much left ... maybe the brownie?' he says, pointing to a dark chocolate square.

'I tell you what, I might try that,' I say, suggesting something lighter-looking.

'What is it?' Fiona asks, as if she's going to count the calories before conceding.

'It looks like some sort of mousse,' I say.

'Well, how about that macaroon thing as well?' she suggests.

I look to the waiter for solidarity: 'Isn't she terrible?' But it's no use; the mousse and macaroon are both put on my plate. What I am learning about Fiona is that she's like Prue Leith: her love of food is founded on giving pleasure to other people. And everything she tells me during our tea together also points to her happiness coming from making other people happy: whether that's giving her own parents grandchildren – which she intimates was more important than having children for herself – or whether it's empowering a woman who has been bullied throughout her marriage to finally stand up to her husband, or whether it's helping an infertile would-be Channel swimmer to eat so she's ready for the sea. It's actually irrelevant whether or not she is a mother, because Fiona Shackleton is mothering. She embodies the verb as much as she embodies the noun. It makes me wonder whether, if I can't be noun, I could be a verb instead.

———

Later, in the pool for one last session before heading to Spain to attempt to complete my six-hour qualifier, I think of the women I've met so far. Some have shown me there are alternative routes to motherhood that can genuinely make you happy; others have made me think about alternative ways of contributing to the world if you can't be a mother. But my conversation with Fiona Shackleton has solidified something else – a thought which started to take form during my conversation with the filmmaker Kim Longinotto at Christmas: there could be ways to mother and make a home without having children.

As I swim, I recall visiting the houses of two of the women on my list of twenty-one: first Frida Kahlo's Blue House in Mexico City (another post-IVF trip) and then Virginia Woolf's Monk's House in Sussex (one sad Sunday on my own). I remember being struck by how both houses were full of vibrant colours, warmth and love, as if they were the homes of happy families, even though neither Kahlo nor Woolf was a mother. Both women had wanted and tried for children but had not been able to have them. In spite of this sadness in their lives, it seemed as if they had decided to be verbs too. It's something to think about as I swim.

Was It Because of the IVF?

Was it because of the IVF, like Fiona said?
Or did it start before that?
Was it because I made you leave the life you had
    to be with me?
Or because I blamed you for the life I left behind
    for you?
Was it because I wanted to have a baby?
Was it because I wanted to have a baby more
    than you did?
Was it because I went on and on about it until
    you looked at me across the dinner table
    and agreed?
But then I couldn't. Was it because of that?
Was it because of the IVF?
The indignity.
The actuation of blame.
The debt.
Was it because I wrote a book about it?
Took my tights off for the *Daily Mail*.
Let Radio 4 come over to our house.

Was it because of that scene you said I'd embellished? The one where we have a row because you've come home drunk the day before our embryos go back.

Was it because I always thought you drank more than you said you did?

Insisted on smelling your breath?

Was it because I could never trust you?

About anything.

Wanted to see your texts and emails.

Never believed what you said to me was true.

Was it because I'm too controlling?

Because I always want my own way.

Was it because I hated it when you wore that leather jacket that I thought made you look old?

Or the time you booked five different restaurants as a surprise for my birthday to be sure there was one that I liked and I didn't want to go to any of them?

Was it because I sometimes got angry and threw stuff?

Was it because I threw your favourite book, the one that you said was really valuable, and it ripped. Was it because of that?

Was it because we stopped having sex for fun?

Because sex became just about having a baby?

Was it because I became completely obsessed with having a baby?

And when it didn't happen, I became obsessed
   with other things instead.
First work, then writing a book, and then
   swimming the Channel.
Was it because I insisted I had to do
   something big?
Was it because I did it to heal me, and didn't
   think about how to heal you?
Was it all this stuff I did to you?

Or was it the stuff you did to me?
Because you did stuff too.
You did.

So We Beat On

I am standing on the beach in Formentera crying. I'm crying because I've done it. I have officially qualified to swim the English Channel by completing six hours in water below sixteen degrees. Every stroke was cold and hard, yet I did it.

And now I am surrounded by the love of people. John and Alice who've been by my side since the beginning when I could hardly manage ten minutes in the water. The lady relayers from Camp Eton who have all become firm friends. Everyone is delighted for me. As am I. But my tears are for other reasons as well. Reasons that will eventually find their words. Until then, I beat on.

Now that I'm a certified contender, the swim ahead feels more frightening than ever. Six hours was hard but the real thing will be more than double that. I don't know that I've got it in me, and I constantly question why I've chosen to take on one of the toughest physical and mental endurance tests on the planet when I've already attempted another one of those eleven times, and it never ended well – once.

I am standing on the beach in Formentera crying. I'm crying because I've done it and the words in my head are the last line of F. Scott Fitzgerald's *The Great Gatsby*. So we beat on. The book that ripped. You, like Jay Gatsby, so difficult to understand. We, boats borne back into the past. I guess I just keep going in the hope that one day I get the chance to swim towards the future. Let this be my chance.

The Chief Constable

'You just have to hang on to it.'

If you're going to stand anyone up for lunch, you wouldn't choose a chief constable. Well, would you? Our introduction had already been unorthodox. I'd sat opposite her at a charity function that I had been invited to by a friend. I hadn't spoken to her; the diameter of the well-dressed table had been too large. But I was fascinated from afar. She looked Amazonian – tall, tanned and commanding – and when I found out she was a police chief it made absolute sense. Following the event, I managed to procure her email address and she agreed to meet me at a hotel in Holborn for lunch. It had been in the diary for months – she's a busy woman. But it was also a crazy time for me at work – the culmination of the capital project I had been working on for years, plus all my Channel training and things being so hard at home – I completely forgot about it until she texted me from the restaurant to ask whether I was coming.

So, yes, I actually stood up Chief Constable Julie Spence, and if you did that you wouldn't expect her to agree to see you again. Well, would you? But she did. She forgave the crime and we set another date. This time for high tea at the Renaissance Hotel in London's St Pancras.

When the waitress comes over to take our order, I insist that Julie lets me buy her a glass of champagne by way of apology for the last time. She concedes, although I find out later she hardly drinks. So her graciousness continues, which is maybe not an adjective you'd imagine you'd use for someone in the police force. But I'm about to find out that there is nothing about Julie Spence that is stereotypical. I ask the waitress whether they do a champagne afternoon tea and when she replies that they do I nod my head at Julie to encourage her that we go for it.

'But can you overdose on the vegetarian sandwiches for me please?' Julie asks politely.

'Do you eat fish?' the waitress enquires.

Julie replies that she will eat a bit of fish but she's not massively keen on it and definitely doesn't like prawns or smoked salmon.

'Whereas I eat everything,' I say to the waitress.

'The eternal hoover,' Julie says.

'I am.'

Julie Spence has the sum of me already. I ask her how long she's been a vegetarian and she says it was just after she got married, which will be twenty-eight years on Saturday. She says it's not a principle thing, just that she never really liked meat.

'I don't know why but it seems strange . . .' I start to say.

She cuts in before I can finish: 'You mean, a vegetarian chief constable?'

'Yes,' I say, grateful to her for saying the crass thing I was thinking.

Then she tells me about a time when she was a sergeant and she was leading some training with a social worker and everybody would joke about the vegetarian police officer and the meat-eating social worker. Julie says the only thing she likes is streaky bacon – crispy, like they do it in the States – and I definitely agree with her on this. Bacon is at its best when it's been cremated.

As we chat, I learn that Julie is no longer a chief constable. She retired from the police in 2010 after thirty-two years of service. She wasn't the first female chief. She was the seventh, which, she tells me, is her lucky number. But I can't help thinking as I start to listen to her life story that she made her luck through sheer 'persistence', which is the word she later gives me for the Channel.

For anyone who is not familiar with the hierarchy of the police, you start as a constable, then become a sergeant, then an inspector, then a chief inspector, then a superintendent, then a chief superintendent, then an assistant chief constable, then a deputy chief constable and finally, a chief constable. Julie started her career at the bottom and got to the top. In fact, she started below the bottom: as a PE teacher. She tells me she loved sport at school and I ask her whether she was a swimmer as she looks like she should be, but she says she was more of a bat and ball girl (howzat?!

Woody Allen, it seems that gym teachers *can* do – they can become chief constables). However, after training to become a teacher, she realised she loved sport but didn't love teaching it, and one cold February morning when she was running up and down the touch line with a tin whistle sticking to her lips, she thought: 'What am I doing here?' So she left and joined the police, which turned out to be a job she loved, but there was nothing about her climb to the top that was easy.

At this point in the conversation our champagne arrives, followed by a selection of sandwiches with an array of different fillings on artisan breads. We cheers and start to tuck in as Julie continues with her story. She tells me that she was the first married woman the police had ever taken and was seen as a bit of a risk as the expectation was that women would do five years, meet a husband and leave. She doesn't say it, but we both know that 'leave' means going off to have a baby. Julie didn't. Obviously, I hadn't known this when I saw her across the table at the charity function, but afterwards I'd turned investigator myself and discovered that she hadn't had children, although she is a stepmother. I wondered what the significance of the insertion of a four-letter word was to motherhood.

'Did you know you didn't want children?' I ask.

'It wasn't that I didn't want but I wasn't avidly pro. I was thinking, if I get my career sorted, maybe I'd have one in my early thirties, but it also coincided with changing husbands.' She picks up a sandwich before continuing: 'I didn't ever really fancy one with my first husband. Maybe if I'd married my current husband first, but he'd already had children. I did give him the option as to whether he'd like more. And he said he didn't want any more nappies and that suited me really. So I do have two stepdaughters and three step-granddaughters.'

Before I can ask her whether she feels like a mother to them she tells me she thinks there were several things that meant she wasn't ultra maternal. The first was having a sister who was eight years younger who she says was left in her charge, which wasn't good for either of them (similar to what the scientist Susan Greenfield had told me about her younger brother); the second was her experience of teaching; and the third, although she recognises it's quite strange for someone in the police, is the fact that she's always been quite squeamish. 'The whole physics thing I couldn't quite get to grips with,' she says. 'Even though people say the pain's fine, I didn't believe them. I thought, there's only a little hole and a great big head . . .'

'So the million-dollar question is,' I say, and then add, ' . . . although it seems very early to come to it over sandwiches . . . have you ever regretted it?'

She ponders for a short while before answering: 'Well, you do often wonder.' And then her thought process seems to change. 'Sometimes I do hate parents who have children as an insurance policy for later in life because I see that going wrong. I see people who hope their children will look after them and it doesn't happen. I think you're just as likely to get comfort from creating friendships as you are from relying on kids. But, I've always wondered,' she says, returning to where she started, 'What if? I've not regretted it but just thought, "What if? How old would they be? What would they look like? What would they be doing?" But then I look at other parents with trials and tribulations and I think I'm well out of it, but I do wonder.'

This seems a good point to ask whether she feels in any way like a mother to her stepdaughters.

'Not really. I was just Julie. I was the one who moderated their father's attitudes and behaviour really. He was quite authoritarian. I tried to get him to relax.'

I tell her I love the idea of the chief constable saying, 'Relax'. She laughs, and this brings the conversation back to her career. When Julie entered the police force there was an expectation that she would rise through the ranks because she was a graduate, but she applied and failed twice to get on the fast-track scheme. Later she was further discouraged when her boss disclosed that her maximum rank potential was considered to be inspector. (i.e. two ranks up from the bottom.) At that point Julie decided to take her career into her own hands. She left the force for two years to broaden her experience by working for the Association of Chief Police Officers, which was responsible for the development of UK policing practices. But when she returned she was overlooked for promotion again. This time her reaction was to do something that many would consider career suicide: she took out an employment tribunal. She says it was a dark time, during which she became known in the force as 'that woman'. But finally, aged forty-three (!), she got the opportunity to go on the Strategic Command Course, which is the gateway to the upper echelons of the police. 'You either get through the eye of that needle or you don't,' she says matter-of-factly. Julie got through, but even then things wouldn't come easy. There are three senior command jobs in the police and you can't leapfrog, you have to go through them all. Julie started as an assistant chief constable and was turned down eighteen times for a deputy chief constable job before she finally got one. Eighteen times – that's seven more 'failures' than my IVF eleven. I can hardly imagine how that must have felt. But Julie is stoical about it, and eventually she did get a deputy job with Cambridgeshire Constabulary. By her own admission, the top job came partly through luck, because her boss dropped himself in some hot water and had to resign, admitting to what he called a 'moment of foolishness'. Julie became acting chief and then got the job in her own right.

I am in awe, unable to find enough superlatives to describe the enormity of what she has achieved.

'You just have to hang on to it,' Julie says. 'That's why I get cross with people who give up. People who fail twice and give up.'

I am astounded by her story and all I can think is that if Julie Spence can get to chief constable after all that, I've got to be able to get across the Channel, even if I fail not once, not twice but eighteen times.

The conversation could have ended there if there hadn't been cakes to come. But they arrive piled high on a stand: warm white scones and an array of jewel-coloured patisseries. It would be a crime not to partake. So we carry on eating and talking. I ask Julie what she's been doing since leaving the force.

'I travel,' she says. 'Since I've retired I've been to forty different countries and I love it.'

'You've been to forty countries in five years?' I gasp.

'About that,' she says. 'Most of it in trail of different wildlife.'

'You love animals?'

'Well, I wouldn't want a dog or a cat in our house, thank you very much,' she says quickly.

'So you don't want a fur baby?'

'Absolutely not. It's just wildlife I love. We've been all the way round Tanzania and Kenya looking at the migration at different points of the year. We've been to the Congo to see lowland gorillas. We've been to Rwanda and Uganda to see other gorillas. We went to Antarctica at Christmas and New Year. We're penguined out. We went to Tasmania and saw the white wallabies and platypus and to Chile for the puma.'

I laugh, baffled and completely charmed by the turn of our conversation and this new side of Julie that has just been revealed. She shows me some photos she's taken, brilliant photos, one with her husband with meerkats on his head and another stunning one of a Pel's fishing owl with huge dark eyes. And then she tells me where they're going next: to Canada to look for spirit bears and then to Zambia for the bat migration; on her future wish list is the Ethiopian wolf and the Arctic belugas. Still laughing and flabbergasted by her list, I tell her that I've always had a dream of visiting every country in the world. 'But so far I think I've been to fewer than you have in the last five years so I better get on with it,' I say.

This reminds me of my conversation at the start of the year with the politician Fiona Mactaggart, who had said you've got to 'carpe diem'. She, and now Julie Spence, had shown me in very different ways how much you can achieve in life if you can't become a mother: you can change the world, you can see the world. You can even do both.

When Julie says goodbye she gives me her card and explains that, like the mantra I am composing for the Channel, she has a little mantra of her own. When she retired someone had called her an inspirational leader, and although her first thought had been: 'Isn't that a description for people like Richard Branson?' she had later decided that if she was an inspirational leader it was purely down to hard work. So she had the following phrase written on her new, post-retirement business card: 'Inspirational leadership needs resilience, persistence and tenacity.' I read the words, which include the one she's given me to take to sea, and there next to them is also a little picture of a lion and a giraffe. I look at former Chief Constable Julie Spence and grin.

Beach Life

The Serpentine Swimming Club may have nurtured more Channel swimmers than any other swimming club in England but most of them will end up in Dover. There is no more revered training ground. Every Saturday and Sunday between the months of May and September, lines of red and yellow hats – emblazoned with Captain Webb's venerable words, 'Nothing great is easy' – can be seen swimming back and forth between the harbour walls. The red hats are the aspiring soloists, the yellow hats are the relayers. And there are other people, in other coloured hats, who are just there for the fun. People joke about Dover. It's not the most salubrious town and the beach is pebbly and the water looks (and sometimes feels) a bit like mud, but it's the spiritual home of Channel swimming and when the sea is full of swimmers training, it's an extraordinary sight.

The harbour is presided over by a larger-than-life bronze bust of Webb, his eyes gazing out towards the horizon. Across the road and in front of him is the beach, and slightly to the right on a line of deckchairs at the back of the shingle, sheltered by the wall of Marine Parade, you will find his chosen apostles: the beach team of Barrie, Irene and Freda, who have dedicated their every summer for many years to making people's Channel dreams come true. You can't miss Barrie: he's the one in the novelty apron or head-to-toe in canary yellow waterproofs when it's raining. Irene is his wife; she's tiny, you could put her in your pocket. And Freda – Freda Streeter – well, she's the General. What she says on the beach goes: ignore it at your peril.

The first time you come down to the beach, like any first day at school, it's intimidating. You don't know the people or the protocol. These, I've found out, are the Dover Beach Rules:

1. Arrive in good time so you're ready to be in the water at 9 a.m.

2. Find a spot for your things. On no account should you put them on top of somebody else's or shift their stuff to the side in order to make room for yours. (I did this once. I saw an opportunity – I thought it was an ample opportunity – to move everything left a little and squeeze my bag in. I didn't make the same mistake again.) If you want a spot for your things alongside the wall that's another reason you need to arrive early. Otherwise be satisfied with the shingle.

3. When you've found your spot and dumped your things, head over to Freda and Irene, who will be sitting next to each other like royalty on deckchair thrones. Freda will ask when your tide is. She'll ask you this every week (don't expect her to remember)

and then she'll give you a time. You won't know how long you're going to be swimming for until this moment. You can put it off for a bit by saying hello to the other swimmers or fiddling with your kit, but eventually you've got to go over. There's no point second-guessing, negotiating or even pleading; what Freda says you do. Irene then writes a number on your hand in thick black marker and writes the same number down on a sheet of paper alongside your name and given time. This is so they can keep track of all the swimmers in the water and make sure everyone stays safe.

4. Now, go back to your spot, get changed and then head to Barrie for greasing. This is the reason for the apron, because he'll also be wielding a vat of yellow sticky stuff which goes under your arms, the straps of your costume, around the groin and along the jaw line (if you're a boy) to stop the chafing.

5. And finally, as you approach the last few minutes before the pain begins, you'll be called to stand in a circle for the General's briefing. She'll tell you to remember to swim outside the red buckets at the end of the breakers so you don't crash into them, and to come in for your first feed on two hours and then every hour after that. Then the General will say that under no circumstances should there be any 'bobbing', which in swimming language means 'standing and talking'. This is the sort of thing I would always get in trouble for as a child.

I don't think I ever had a school report that didn't read: 'Jessica would do much better if she spent more time concentrating on her work and less time chatting to her friends.' But down in Dover I've changed the habit of a lifetime, because as far as I'm concerned bobbing is even worse than swimming. All that happens when you stand and chat is that you get cold, and given you're not allowed to get out until your allotted time is up, it's not worth it as it only adds agony to agony.

So those are the beach rules. You'll know them now if you ever want to swim the Channel or find yourself in Dover one weekend waiting for the ferry and wondering what on earth is going on. Strangers to the town often lean over the railings along the promenade and ask what everyone is doing, and then nod in admiration when they're told the hats in the water are training to swim the English Channel. Most people get the magnitude of this, but apparently a guy came down one day adamant he wanted to try and swim to France there and then. Sometimes it does looks quite close, so if it's a nice day and you fancy yourself a good swimmer, I guess you might think it's possible. Occasionally, even I look across and think it doesn't look too far, but given it takes me an hour to swim out to the red bucket on the right, down to the harbour wall on the east and then back to the bucket and into the beach, I know it isn't.

If the conditions are bad, Freda forbids you from swimming to the harbour wall; you can only go as far as the long groyne, known to the swimmers as 'slopey', or sometimes only as far as the short groyne, known as 'stumpy'. I like stumpy and slopey, they provide the perfect frame to the Premier Inn, which has become my Dover hotel of choice on Saturday nights. When I swim between them I breathe wistfully towards its purple insignia and dream of the bath I'll be having later. Lying like Cleopatra in the hotel bath after a long training session has become my paradise. It's on a par with all the food I get to consume after. During training food is largely limited to liquid carbohydrate and jelly babies, which are the staple of Channel swimming because they're sweet and easily digestible. I may not have a real baby but these days ones made of gelatine and sugar are in plentiful supply. Like animals at the zoo, we come into the shore on feeding time and hold out our paws gratefully for half a cup of warmth and two jellied jewels. Later on we might get a piece of banana. I've always liked my bananas green with the pointy ends cut off neatly but these days I devour a browning stump as if it's Michelin-starred. And if you're doing a really long swim you might even get treated with a chocolate mini roll or a Milky Way towards the end, which is ecstasy. The small edible things in my life have become symbols of joy and the large edible things I get to have afterwards are guilt-free jubilation.

But I digress. The point I'm trying to make is that the swim up and then down Dover harbour feels like the longest two lengths I've ever done in my life. So if that man thought he could swim the Channel there and then, in fact if anyone thinks that the Channel is just a little strip of water that you can pop across, just put them in the harbour under the watchful gaze of Captain Matthew Webb and his apostles, and tell them to swim. Then they'll see.

The General

'Eventually your tits will scrape the sand.'

When I had lunch with Jackie Cobell, my Ice Queen Foster Mother, I asked her what she thought of Freda Streeter, the legendary Channel swimming trainer. Jackie said that she makes grown men cry, and if you're not up to it she'll tell you. I've already said that what Freda says goes and this is exactly why. She's seventy-six years old, has been on the beach for over thirty years and has seen it all. If anyone knows what it takes to be a Channel swimmer, Freda does. And not because she's swum it herself. If you ask her she'll say: 'Mate, there's a ferry over there, a plane up there and if you listen hard a train down there. Why would I want to?' But she knows because she's trained more Channel swimmers than anyone in the world, including her daughter, Alison Streeter, who has swum it a staggering forty-three times, which is more than anyone else. Ever.

Now I just have to add an aside here, which is that swimming the English Channel forty-three times is not normal. I repeat: NOT NORMAL. Someone once said to me, and I think this is the only way to comprehend it, that

Alison is half-human, half-seal. She has achieved the most extraordinary feats of human endurance that quite possibly will never be matched. And along with herself there is only one other common denominator in her achievements – her mother.

About two weeks into Dover training, I sidled up to Freda, who hardly knew me from the other swimmers on the beach, and asked if I could interview her about motherhood. Just asking the question made me nervous as I wasn't sure how she'd respond and I didn't want to do anything that would make her take against me so early in the season. But she said yes and invited me to her home in Surrey one evening.

Freda lives alone: her husband, Alan, died a few years ago. When I arrive, we start by feeding the fish. She has a pond in her back garden packed with koi carp, which somehow seems apt. Then we take the washing in and I notice that sitting on the floor by the back door are a couple of vats of Barrie's yellow grease, which she tells me she mixes to her own recipe. After that we sit in the garden for a bit so she can have a fag. Then we go inside and she makes cheese, ham and tomato panini and puts one on a plate for her, and two on a plate for me. She adds a couple of spring onions on the side. And even though I protest (a bit) at being given two panini and I'm not that keen on spring onions, I know I'm going to eat it all because I want to please her.

'So where do you want to start?' she asks directly.

There's so much I want to know, but it seems right to start with Alison's story. Freda begins by telling me she was never a swimmer when she was young as life was a struggle after the war. She was married at twenty-two and became a wages clerk for the electrical company Philips. Then one day someone came to recruit people to help teach disabled children to swim and Freda thought she'd give it a go. She loved doing it so much that she decided to qualify as a swimming teacher and so her three children – Alison, Karl and Neil – grew up around the poolside. Then when Alison was seven years old she developed severe asthma and they were told by doctors that the best way to help it was for her to sing, row or swim.

'Well, if you've heard her sing, mate, that was out of the question,' Freda says. 'And where do you get a seven-year-old to learn to row? But she could swim so we thought maybe it's time we got her in a club. And she took off. Then Karl, we put him in and he was good. But Neil, he was just amazing. If Neil had had the mental ability to stick at it like the others did he would have made team GB easy. I can tell you now, at thirteen years old he was doing something like 58 seconds for 100 front crawl, 1 minute 5 for 100 fly and 1 minute 10 for 100 back, but he had such a good breaststroke too he was only doing about 1 minute 13 for that. But he didn't want to do it.'

I listen to her, captivated by her ability to reel off these times and know how fast her son swam over thirty years ago, and then ask what changed.

'Well, we took him to the Surrey championships one night. He was swimming in the junior 200 metres and he qualified for the final, nine seconds faster than anyone else.

I said: "Well done, son, that's yours in the final now." And he goes: "What do you mean?" So I go: "Well you're nine seconds faster than anyone else. If you swim it again, mate, it's gonna be yours," and he goes: "I ain't swimming that again for a hunk of metal.'"

'So he didn't do it?' I say, gripped by the drama.

'He swam it, but like a plonker. He just wasn't interested.'

'So did that upset you?'

'No. I never forced them to swim. Never. I did force them to train because, living around here, there was a whole group of kids they would have got into so much trouble together, so I made sure they were worn out before we got back home so they couldn't.'

'And then there was Alison,' I say.

'Well, the rest is history,' she replies.

That history started when Alison was fourteen and broke the junior and senior records for swimming the Solent. She then went on to swim the English Channel aged eighteen. The following year she did a two-way crossing (there and back) and she was the first ever woman to swim it three ways (there, back and there again). She was also the first woman to swim the North Channel from Ireland to Scotland (not as famous as the English Channel but even harder on account of the fact it's colder and there are nastier jellyfish). In fact, throughout her swimming career Alison has trampled over existing records by being the first or the fastest countless times. She has swum all over the world and has swum the English Channel more than anyone in the world, earning her the title of Queen of the Channel,

Member of the Most Excellent Order of the British Empire (MBE).[3]

It was only after Alison's two-way crossing, at the age of just nineteen, that people started to realise what a phenomenon she was. 'Everybody in the world, and I mean everybody in the world, sat up and said, "Where did that come from? Who are you?"' Freda says. 'And it hit the press big time. Real big time.'

She tells me how Alison had decided to raise money in memory of a little boy they knew who had died of leukaemia and when she set off to do the two-way she'd raised about a thousand pounds, but by the time she'd finished thousands more had come in. When she tells me this I think of my businesswoman, Nicola Horlick, whose daughter Georgie had leukaemia and who, albeit unconsciously, Alison had been swimming to help. Sometimes it seems as if the women in my story are linked by an invisible thread.

During our conversation I ask Freda several times if she's proud of Alison and I can't help noticing that she continually bats the question away with another answer entirely. There's something that tells me she's not a conventional pushy mother seeking glory in her children's achievements. Her psychology is much more complex than this. It's almost as if her role as Alison's coach is separate from her role as Alison's mother, and when I ask Freda what she thinks her own greatest achievement has been, she says it's all her swimmers that succeed, not singling any of them out. She tells me it's what makes all those wet windy days on the beach worth it, and when they achieve their dreams she's got what she wants, the score's settled.

Perhaps Freda is the sort of woman that Camila Batmanghelidjh had said the Western world hadn't yet fully found a way of describing: someone who is less driven by her own personal need and more by a vocation to help others. It just happens that Freda is also a mother. In fact, she's the mother of one of the most successful open-water swimmers in the world. I think you can call that karma.

Suddenly there's a sound from the kitchen and we both start.

'What's that?' I say.

'I think it might have been the fridge,' Freda replies, but admits to being a little bit jumpy because there has recently been a spate of break-ins in the area.

'I don't think anyone's going to steal the grease, but let's have a look,' I say.

We go into the kitchen; no one's there, but the getting up provides the impetus to go outside for Freda to have a fag. This time we sit at the front on the side wall.

'So how do you know the ones who are going to do it, Freda?' I ask.

'Jessica,' she says, 'I've not been around swimmers for as long as I have . . . don't ask me how I know.'

'You just know?' I finish what I think she's about to say.

'Yeah.'

'But what is it?'

'If I knew, I could tell you.'

'So at what point do you know if they're going to do it or not?'

She sighs: 'Possibly quite early on in the training.'

'Yeah?' My voice sounds worried, as if she might have already made an assessment of me. She tells me that the giveaway is often the people who take a long time getting into the water, as well as the people who get out early.

After a moment's pause taking this in, two words escape involuntarily from my mouth: 'I'm scared . . .'

'What are you scared of?' she asks, turning to look at me squarely.

'I'm scared of . . .' I break off in the same way I did when I said exactly this to Jackie, as if I don't really know how to articulate what I'm feeling, and Freda immediately repeats what Jackie said to me: 'You're scared about failing.'

'Yeah.'

But I know there's something more I need to say, because my fear is far bigger than whether or not I can do it. I'm just as afraid, maybe more so, of the things out of my control that will stop me. Nature's let me down too many times already and I don't trust her not to disappoint me again. Then, as if Freda can see what's inside my head she says suddenly: 'My best bet is always that tree down there,' she points towards her neighbour's back garden.

'Why? What does it tell you?' I ask.

'I sit and watch that tree and I know by how it's behaving what the sea's like. Just by the way it rustles.'

'That's what I'm scared of,' I say. 'The sea. What if it turns and I've got no choice but to get out? Or what if someone else decides I'm not going to make it – because I'm too slow or something.'

'Who's your pilot?'

'Paul. On *Optimist*.'

'Paul won't take you out because you're slow. Paul will just tell you to get your arse into gear.'

I don't say that my arse can only go in first gear.

'Trouble is,' she says, 'you're all sitting there thinking, "Christ, it's twenty-one miles, it's this, it's that." Forget it. When your swim comes you get on the beach, and for crying out loud don't think you're going to swim to France, don't even put it there, mate!' – she points to her head and taps it twice – 'it's too much for the brain to take. What's going to happen is, you stand on the beach and they give you the signal and you start to swim. And you swim to your first feed. You take your first feed, you never ask them on the boat how far you've gone, you never ask them how much longer, and then they can't tell you any lies. You don't want to know anyway. Feed as quick as you can and get going. Just a quick conversation so they know you're OK and compos mentis. Apart from that you swim to the next feed, and you keep swimming to the next feed, and you keep your arms and legs moving as if you're the boat's third engine, and if you keep your arms and legs moving, take your drink, go quick, eventually – well, eventually your tits will scrape the sand.'

I laugh. She stubs out her cigarette and then we go back inside to finish our panini and spring onions.

'Freda, I'm asking everyone I meet to give me a word for my Channel swim. Will you give me one?'

'Well, my favourite word is "if",' she says.

'If,' I say, in admiration at the poetry of her choice.

'Yes, if,' she says again. 'The smallest word in the English language with the biggest meaning.'

There's a moment of silence.

'Mind you, I already don't like your sayings – what if the weather blows up, what if I get pulled out, what if, what if, what if. You, Jessica, you've got to remember what I've said. Just take each drink as it comes.'

I wonder what might happen if I could do that. If I could just take each drink as it comes all the way to France.

'They're not very nice those onions, are they. They're a bit chewy,' Freda says.

I pick one up and take a bite. 'They're fine,' I reply. Just like a child who wants to do nothing more than make her swimming mother proud.

Gertrude Ederle

When Alison Streeter first hit the headlines for swimming from England to France and back again, she was the same age the American Gertrude Ederle was when she became the first woman to swim the Channel – just nineteen.

Ederle also became an overnight sensation. The race to become the first woman to cross the English Channel had captured the imagination of the world press, and in the summer of 1926 several women had it in their sights. Ederle's rivals included another American, Mille Gade, who made newspaper headlines for being 'the first mother to attempt to conquer the Channel'. In an interview she was quoted as saying: 'I think no woman is at her best physically or otherwise until she is a mother.'* I admire Gade – she was trying to challenge preconceptions. But comments such as these have long encouraged the division of women by their desire and ability to reproduce, reinforcing the

---

* Mille Gade interviewed in Pennsylvania's *Clearfield Progress*, 24 August 1925.

stigma that comes with childlessness, whether chosen or circumstantial. Whereas men are never pitted against each on the basis of fatherhood.

Ederle's first attempt at crossing the Channel in 1925 had failed when she was pulled out of the water against her wishes. But the following year she was back, and on 6 August 1926, at seven in the morning, Ederle walked into the waves at Cap Gris-Nez in France. Her last words to her father were: 'Don't let anyone take me out unless I ask.' She was covered in grease and wearing a daring (for the times) two-piece costume, with an American flag sewn on the front. Within minutes of starting out she had a series of severe stomach cramps and later said that she regretted the peach she had eaten earlier. But the pain subsided and she was soon swimming at an excellent stroke rate.

A few hours out from the coast the sea started to stir and the sky turned gunmetal grey. Then it began to rain, and the wind whipped up the waves. Fears began to spread on her support boat that if the weather continued like this she didn't stand a chance of making it. Even Gertrude herself, who had been so confident at the beginning that the English coast was eminently reachable, could now see it receding. However, she resolved to put her head down and not look up and just carry on swimming for as long as she could keep alive. Her trainer, Bill Burgess, who had become the second man to swim the Channel on his sixteenth attempt, was deeply concerned that she was swimming to her death. He confronted Ederle's father, insisting that she be taken out of the water before the waves battered her into unconsciousness. But Gertrude's father kept the promise he'd made to his daughter on the beach. She battled on, the tide doing its best to drag her past Dover and towards Folkestone, and if it had its way into the Atlantic and back home to New York. Gertrude's sister, Margaret, who was on the support boat, could see her sibling was in a lot of physical pain, but she was less concerned about the battering to her body and more worried about whether her sister had the mental strength to continue in the conditions. This was the biggest test of her nineteen-year-old life. But Ederle did what Freda Streeter would later counsel her daughter and all her Channel children to do. She concentrated on the small strip of water in front of her, and when she'd swum that she swam it again.

And then the Channel did what only the Channel can decide to do. It turned the tide back in her favour, cleared the skies, and suddenly, it looked like she had a chance of making it. It was just after nine in the evening when Gertrude allowed herself to look up. She'd been swimming for over fourteen hours. Through the darkness she could see bonfires blazing on the beach ahead, lit by the crowds gathering there. It was the sign she needed to make her final push. People had poured into Kingsdown, just east of Dover, to see her come ashore. As she stumbled out of the waves they reached out and touched her head and her hands as if she was some sort of messiah, and when she returned to America thousands upon thousands of people lined the streets of Manhattan to honour her with a ticker-tape parade.

That day in August 1926, Gertrude Ederle made history not only for becoming the first woman to swim the English Channel, but for doing it in just fourteen hours and thirty-nine minutes – two hours faster than the fastest of the five men who had preceded her, and seven hours faster than Captain Webb (although he was a breaststroker, whereas Ederle was a proponent of the modern crawl). It was a seminal moment in the world's move towards acceptance that women could really be equal to men. Gertrude Ederle had shattered the myth of women being the weaker sex. When the mayor of New York presented her with a scroll of honour he said, 'When history records the great crossings, they will speak of Moses crossing the Red Sea, Caesar crossing the Rubicon and Washington crossing the Delaware, but frankly, Gertrude Ederle, your crossing of the British Channel must take its place alongside of these.'

Less than two years after Ederle swam the Channel, her hearing started to deteriorate. It had been bad since childhood due to a bout of measles but got worse as a result of the amount of time she had spent in the water. A year after this she was arrested for failing to appear in court for a speeding offence. She pleaded guilty, claiming the reason for her speed was that she was late for an appointment with her audiologist. Her hearing had got so bad that the magistrate had to stand right next to her and shout into her ear that he was passing a suspended sentence. After the trial she joked with reporters that the worst thing about her condition was not being able to hear the nice things her beau said to her. Gertrude had fallen in love and was engaged to be married –

but later the same year, when she allegedly acknowledged to her fiancé that her hearing problems must be hard to live with, he agreed and promptly left her. Ederle was devastated and would remain single for the rest of her life. She said once that, although she was proud of swimming the Channel, if she'd known she would lose her hearing because of it she might never have done it.

A few years later things got even worse for Ederle. She fell down some stairs and was seriously injured. The prognosis at the time was that she would never walk or swim again, but using the determination she'd shown in the Channel, she decided to prove her doctors wrong. Over a period of many months, she rehabilitated herself, and on the thirteenth anniversary of her Channel crossing – 6 August 1939 – she swam one length of a swimming pool in New York in front of an invited audience who clapped and cheered as she reached the end. There is no more poignant image of how far she had fallen and how far she had come. She spent the latter part of her life teaching deaf and disabled children to swim.

Gertrude Ederle died on 30 November 2003 at the age of ninety-eight. Sadly, she never escaped the image of the girl who, at nineteen, became the most famous and celebrated woman in the world and then lost it all. During the course of her life people gradually forgot who she was and she is little remembered today – there is no bust of her at Dover harbour alongside Captain Webb's. But Gertrude Ederle did something big for women that should never be forgotten; that's why she deserves her place on my list of twenty-one.

And what of Mille Gade? Well, less than a month later she too made it across, becoming the second woman to conquer the Channel. She didn't beat Ederle's time, but she made headlines around the world as the first mother to swim it. Ederle told the crowds in New York that she had swum the Channel for 'America'; Gade said, 'I swam for my two children and their future.'

———————

My tide and time is getting close now. Last week I received an email from Serpentine Nick:

> *Jessica,*
> *People swim the Channel for all sorts of reasons. It's all about the strength of the things deep inside you that are driving you forward, as those are the things you'll have to call upon in the dark times. Wishy-washy motivations just don't work when the chips are down. Work out WHY you really want to do this, and get that clear in your head.*
> *Nick*

Mille Gade swam the Channel for her children. I'm swimming it for me and Gertrude Ederle and the children we never had.

The Gateway Woman

'The answer to life is to live the question.'

I've found a woman who has written the manual to living life without the children you always wanted. Now I don't have to write it, and can focus on my manual to swimming the Channel. Her name is Jody Day. I first read about her in the Sunday papers. She's the founder of Gateway Women, an online social network for people who are involuntarily childless. She has also written a book called *Living the Life Unexpected: 12 Weeks to Your Plan B for a Meaningful and Fulfilling Future Without Children.* I wish I'd found her sooner, because this Channel thing has taken way longer than twelve weeks.

Jody agrees to meet me for lunch at a chichi private members' club in Chiswick, not far from where I work and she lives. I'm not a member; I've blagged the two of us in. Last time I was here I was with a friend who is a member, and I made the mistake of ordering a club sandwich without looking closely enough at the ingredients on the menu. It came with egg. Do club sandwiches usually come with egg? If they do, they shouldn't. Chicken and egg in the same dish is just wrong: you can't have a mother and her baby on the same plate. Anyway, I'm not making that mistake again. Today I order risotto and Jody orders shepherd's pie. As we're waiting for our meal to arrive, I explain that I'm setting off for my Channel swim in a few weeks and that by the time I reach France – if I reach France – I'm hoping I'll have found the answer to the question: does motherhood make you happy?

In return Jody tells me her story. It's different from mine but there are some similarities. She got married in her twenties and then in her early thirties she and her husband started trying for a baby but didn't fall pregnant. They underwent all the routine fertility tests, were given an 'unexplained' diagnosis – just like ours – and were about to undergo IVF. But during the years of trying to conceive their relationship had started to break down. Jody says she distinctly remembers being in the bath one day and thinking she couldn't go through with the fertility treatment. She describes it as a tough moment but also a very maternal one – she just knew it was wrong to bring a baby into a relationship that was imploding. She and her husband separated and she hoped she'd meet someone else to have a family with. She was confident that when she did they could just 'do IVF' and make it happen, although she knows now that it isn't the magic bullet so many people think it is. But, aged forty-three (!), she was still alone and realised she'd run out of time. Setting up Gateway Women was her version of doing something big. She says it saved her, like I'm hoping the Channel will save me.

'So, can I ask, when you hear the word "mother", what's the first thing that comes into your head?' I say.

She ponders on my question for a few seconds: 'I think the word that comes up for me is "conflict",' she replies. 'I think our society's relationship with motherhood is conflicted – whether you're a mother or not. I've met so many women now who are deeply traumatised about not being able to be mothers and society makes judgements on them because of it.'

Jody's words echo everything I know but, listening to them, I also have a sudden epiphany. 'Actually, you know what I've learned from all the women I've met?' I say. 'I've learned that whether you have a child or not, most people need something else as well.'

'But a lot of women think a child is the answer,' Jody says.

'Yeah, and then they realise it isn't.'

'And they're now a domestic servant with a full-time caring job and there are twenty years until shift's over,' Jody replies, and then says she thinks this is the other side of the conflict, because mothers are allowed to admit it to each other but when they're talking to 'civilians' they've got to say it's the most meaningful and wonderful thing they've ever done – unless you're the filmmaker Kim Longinotto, of course. What annoys Jody is that most people don't tell the whole story. This often makes childless women feel like they're missing out: 'Motherhood may well be wonderful, but the story that the media sells, and that the mothers who are not being completely honest sell, is not the answer,' she says. 'It's another messy imperfect human experience; it's just a different one to the one I'm having. I no longer believe I am a lesser person because I'm not a mother, but I did. I thought my life was worthless, I thought I might as well just leave.'

'So are you left with any sadness about not having children?' I ask.

'My experience is that I'm through my grief but it will always be a scar on my heart,' she replies. 'What happens for me is the experiences of grief are further apart and I recover from them quicker. But usually it's a new aspect of my loss that I haven't encountered or thought about before that gets me. For example, a friend recently had a baby and I was pretty sure grief would come up and I was waiting for it. But I was really surprised what it was. I left a message on her voicemail, congratulating her on the birth. And when I put the phone down I thought: no one is ever going to leave me a message like that. And then I thought: oh, now it comes. I've learned to live with those moments and actually kind of treasure them because they're the echoes of love I had for my children. You only grieve what you have loved. I loved my children, I just didn't meet them.'

I'm hushed for a moment by her wisdom, and then suggest we order pudding. Chocolate tart for me, Eton mess for her. I like a woman who can do pudding at lunch.

'So,' Jody says, 'you've now interviewed all these women, do you know what your answer is going to be when you reach France?'

I'm taken aback. No one has asked me this so directly before, but my swim is imminent; these meetings must come to an end soon. 'I don't know,' I falter. 'I've learned so many things, but I'm not sure I do know the answer . . . yet.'

'Well, there's a quote from the Austrian writer Rilke which you might like,' she offers. 'It's in his letters to a young poet and I can't quite remember the exact words but he says something like: "The answer to life is to live the question."'

'That's beautiful,' I say and then repeat the words back. 'My answer is to keep living the question.' I nod and smile: 'I think that might be it.'

At the end of our lunch together, the word the Gateway Woman Jody Day gives me is 'mystery,' and after we say goodbye I count up all the words I've been given so far by the women I've met. I have twenty in total. I decide I need just one more: twenty-one words from twenty-one women for my twenty-one miles to happiness which in the end might not be a beach or even a baby, it might just be a life of living this mysterious question.

The Seven and Six

Serpentine Boris said to me the other day: 'It's not the getting there that changes you, it's the training.'

If that's right, the day the training truly changed me was Saturday 18 July. Or maybe it was Sunday 19 July. Actually, it was both these days: Saturday 18 and Sunday 19 of July – the weekend when I first completed the legendary 'seven and six', the pinnacle of Channel swimming training, in Dover harbour.

Like a marathon, when you're training to swim the Channel you're not expected to have done the whole distance before you actually do it. The general rule of thumb is that on the big day you can increase considerably what you've done beforehand. Adrenaline gets you through, along with the knowledge that this is the culmination of everything you've been working towards, so you can give it every last bit of energy you've got. To qualify to swim the Channel you need to prove you can do six hours in water below sixteen degrees, but to really show the Dover beach team you've got what it takes you need to do the seven and six: seven hours in the harbour on Saturday, six hours on Sunday – a total of thirteen hours of swimming in one weekend. The killer bit is getting out on Saturday and going to sleep knowing that you've got to get up the next day and do it all (minus one hour) over again. I was dreading it. I think everyone dreads it. If you didn't dread it, you wouldn't be giving it the respect it deserves.

You know it's coming but because of the way things work on the beach, you don't know when. Two weeks before, General Freda had given me a 'four and four'. That had been a surprise: it was less than I had done the previous weekend and less than I had been bracing myself for on the way down to Dover. I guess it should have been a pleasant surprise, but when you know what's waiting there's part of you that wants to get it over and done with. The not knowing what you're going to have to swim each weekend is really tough. You can't prepare yourself mentally. But I know that's part of the training; you don't know what the Channel is going to throw at you, so you need to be ready for everything and nothing.

The weekend after the four and four, Freda gives me a six and four. On the Saturday morning, Chris (doubting Coniston Chris) is down in Dover. He's half the size he was last year, having lost all his Channel weight, and tells me that this season he's struggling to stay in very long because he gets too cold. But he's got nothing to prove; he's already done it. Of course he did it.

'What have you been given today?' he asks – the question on everyone's lips first thing on Saturday and Sunday mornings.

'Six,' I say. 'Can you believe it, Chris? Six! Me!'

'No,' he says bluntly. 'When I met you, I didn't think you stood a god in hell's chance of getting to France.'

I laugh. I don't mind his doubting me. Everyone doubted me. In some ways it's harder now that they're not doubting me as much as they did. Although I know they do still doubt me a bit. I continue to complain incessantly about every hour in the water. Despite all my eating I haven't seemed to put on much weight because of all the exercise so I'm still struggling with the cold. I tell anyone who will listen how hard it is and how much I hate it. I stalk people to swim with to help me get through. But nearly everyone is faster than me; either that or they're hiding from the pessimist because positivity is generally considered to be the mindset of choice on the beach. I know they see my negativity as my noose.

'The thing is, Chris,' I say, 'what you didn't realise is that I have a secret weapon.'

'What's that?' He sounds interested.

I tap my head. 'This. This is my secret weapon. What's in here.'

I leave it at that. I don't say what I'm thinking, which is that you don't get through eleven rounds of unsuccessful IVF if you're not made of something strong. And I guess one of the things I would like the world to know is that going through infertility and IVF is so tough that it can even turn a non-swimming, cold-hating, exercise-loathing pessimist into a Channel contender.

So on Saturday 18 July, Freda finally gives me the number; Irene writes in black marker on my hand; Barrie, in his apron, greases me up and says: 'Go on, Jessie, you can do it.' After two hours I come in for feeding time with all the other animals in this zoo, and then each hour again after that. When I swim past the Premier Inn I breathe left towards it and think: 'Looking forward to seeing you later.' I can't wait for my bath, then food and my 'guaranteed good night's sleep', which cannot be guaranteed when doing the seven and six because how can you sleep when you know that tomorrow you've got to get up and do it all over again (minus one)?

And on Sunday 19 July, Freda gives me the number; Irene writes in black marker on my hand; Barrie, in his apron, greases me up and says: 'Go on, Jessie, you can do it.' After two hours I come in for feeding time with the others, and then each hour again after that. When I swim past the Premier Inn I think: 'I love you: your bath; your food; your "guaranteed good night's sleep", which cannot be guaranteed . . . but don't worry, I'll be back next week to do it again.'

It's true. The training has changed me and, afterwards, when we're all walking to the station, homebound, someone remarks on how happy I look, my face aglow, stripy white and brown, hat-marked after thirteen hours of swimming. I say that I am: I'm so happy to be on solid ground. And as I lean back into my seat on the train to London, exhausted, I declare: 'I can't believe I did it. I'm not even an open-water swimmer.' And in unison, everyone around me says: 'You are now!'

Ten Minutes

When they ask me what's the longest I've swum for, I already know what I'll say. I don't know who they are – some as-yet-unknown third person plural – but I know I'll say that the longest I've swum for is ten minutes.

The first ten minutes in cold water is the worst. I don't think I'll ever stop dreading the moment it hits my inner skin. Nevertheless, I never hang around on the side of the lake or the shoreline. Delaying this moment is pointless; fear of the cold never gets better until you get in – or you turn back and decide that you're not getting in at all, but I can't allow myself to ever think that. In the immortal words of Margaret Thatcher, this lady's not for turning; so you turn if you want to, but for me it isn't an option.

After the first few strokes, your heart heaving, it does get better; you might even experience a moment of joy. Being outside in natural water is, for at least one second, a wonderful thing. Savour it: it might only be a second, and you're only one minute in. Head down and the cold rushes over you; getting your body wet is the first thing, your head the nerve-wracking next as you feel those first sensations of cold-water shock all over again. I remember as a child going to swim in the Parliament Hill Lido on Hampstead Heath and a man running out of the changing room and bombing himself in. My dad, who wasn't a person generally prone to giving worldly advice, told me that this was stupid. He said that if the man wasn't used to the cold the shock to his body, and especially his head, could be fatal. It's funny the things we remember, and all the things we forget. But I remember my dad saying this and I've carried it with me until now. So I never dive in. I glide into the water. I don't stop to rethink it, I keep going, slowly and steadily: walk – cold – body under – cold – second of joy (maybe) – cold – head down – cold – one minute gone – cold – nine minutes to go – still cold.

The thing about ten minutes in cold open water is that it feels like an hour – it should be counted in sextupled time. I suppose if you're just swimming for fun (weird, but some people do), then the fact that ten minutes equals an hour could be seen as a bonus, as it means that you can get your daily dose of exercise over and done with quickly. Sadly, for me, ten minutes is just the start, and the only way I can get through it is by not looking at my watch. But I have to wear a watch – it's like a safety blanket in case I get desperate – yet I try my best never to look at it because seeing that I've only done ten minutes when it feels like I've been in for an hour is something I try to avoid.

So the first ten minutes is the worst, comparable only to the last. However long I've swum for, however long I've managed not to look at my watch, there will come a moment when I finally give in and glance at my wrist. Generally speaking, it's always a disappointment and there's longer to go than I hoped. Head down – swim on – swim on longer before I dare to look again. But eventually the last ten minutes does come. I feel a rush of relief. Dover beach beckons, along with inane happiness at the prospect of my feet being back on dry land. But the problem with the final ten minutes is that once I've allowed myself to give in to it, I can't stop looking at my watch and the seconds pass interminably. If I'm near the beach I swim towards it in the vain hope that when I get there it will be time to get out, but it never is and I have to swim out to the first red bucket again and then back. The only way to get through it is to keep telling myself: just ten minutes and then and then and then the end.

So when they ask me what's the longest I've swum for, I already know what I'll say. It wasn't Coniston. It wasn't my six-hour qualifier in Formentera. It wasn't my first seven and six in Dover. It won't even be whatever is still to come. When they ask me, I'll say the longest I've ever swum for is ten minutes.

Dad and Mum

'I don't think you can call children an achievement.
They're what you've been given.'

My tide opens next week. Paul, my pilot, calls to check that I'm ready to go.

'Have you got your support crew in place?' he asks.

I tell him that John will be leading the team.

'Parents coming?'

'No.'

'That's good. Parents are never a good idea. They don't like seeing their children in pain.'

I don't mention that I've been hiding my pain from them for a long time in order to protect them from theirs. I'm good at it.

'Partner?' Paul asks.

'Yes.'

'Is he coming?' Paul reframes the question.

'I hope so, I'm not sure.'

And then, as if pilots are as sensitive to subtext as they are to the sea, he says: 'I had a swimmer once, when he got across first thing he said when he got back on the boat was: "Relationships come and go but I'll always have the Channel."'

For the rest of the day I think about Paul's words. That man was right: there's no guarantee that people will stay with you – parents, partners or even your children. But if you swim from England to France, you'll always be a Channel swimmer. No one can ever take that away.

——————

My dad will never know I went through eleven rounds of IVF trying to become a mother. He'll never know I wrote a book about it. He'll never know that on the day he died, I had taken a pregnancy test in the morning, after our tenth round of treatment, and that it was negative. We had every reason to be hopeful. It was the first round at a new clinic and we'd done some things differently and our embryos had achieved a 100 per cent fertilisation rate. It was the highest fertilisation rate we'd ever had, and according to the embryologist they were all top quality.

I knew dad was dying. He was ninety-two and in the previous few years he'd suffered a series of strokes. He'd hung on for as long as he could, but he was ready to go. On that tenth round of IVF I allowed myself to believe that the circle of life was more than a great song from *The Lion King*. But it wasn't. Of that day, I wrote: 'Life gives and it takes away. Today it took away a lot and gave me nothing back in return.' My dad will never read those words.

He would have been proud of me becoming a writer,

prouder, I think, than of me becoming a mother. My dad's mother was a writer, but she struggled to find her voice at a time when women were expected to be wives and mothers, not poets. That's certainly what her husband, my grandfather, expected, and he had her consigned to an asylum when she disobeyed. Her struggle led to her suicide. No one should have to find their mother hanging from the door frame in her bedroom, but my father did.

My mum knows I went through eleven rounds of IVF, although she didn't know at the time. I wanted to protect her from my disappointment as well as her own. But she knows now because she's read my book about it. I remember her calling me when I was hurtling down the stairs from our flat on my way to work. I was late. The phone rang. I picked up and said 'hello' and I knew immediately from the way that my Mum said 'hello' back that she'd read it. I know it was hard for her. But I also believe that writing about my pursuit of motherhood and the darkness it took me into made it easier to live with. I don't know why, but it has, and I'd urge anyone to try it, about anything in their life that hurts and they are keeping secret. Get it out – say it; write about it; sing about it; paint about it; do anything you want about it – but I promise that something that seems so all-consuming inside of you will become much smaller when you let it meet the world. It will be easier to live with, not just for you but for everyone around you.

———

My dad would have been in awe of me even attempting to swim the Channel. My mum, like mums are wont to be, is just worried. A week before my tide opens, I go round to see her.

'Mum?'

'Yes.'

'I've got these questions I've been asking the women I've been meeting. Would you mind if I asked you some of them?'

'OK,' she says, but she looks nervous. I can tell the white noise is loud in her head. I think she thinks the questions are going to test her general knowledge and she won't know the answers. She doesn't want to look foolish.

'What have been the biggest achievements of your life so far, Mum?'

She doesn't say anything immediately. I can tell she's relieved it's not Trivial Pursuit but she still doesn't know how to answer. She's silent for a long time, thinking about it.

'I don't think I've achieved very much at all,' she says eventually. 'You'll have to give me more time to think about it.'

'What about having two children?' I suggest.

'I don't think you can call children an achievement. They're what you've been given,' she says.

I put my hand over hers in silent connection.

'Well, what's happiness to you then, Mum?'

She thinks again: 'I'm not interested in happiness for myself. If I can make other people happy then I feel happy.'

Her answer reminds me of some of the women I've met who seem to derive their happiness partly or wholly from giving it away. Yet I am also aware that over this last extraordinary year of my life I have only met these women once, so everything I've seen of them and said about them can only be an impression. I don't really know them. But I do know my mum. I've known her for over forty-three years. I know that she's speaking the truth when she says this.

'Do you think motherhood makes you happy, Mum?'

'I think it's a desire that is natural to a woman and provides tremendous fulfilment,' she says, and then finishes her sentence with an afterthought: 'If you are fortunate enough to have a child, of course.'

It doesn't hurt me when she says this because it's the truth. We don't have to hide that from each other any more.

'And how would you like to be remembered, Mum?'

'That I've been a good mother.'

I look at her. I feel emotion welling. I try to push it down as I've always tried to push my true feelings down, in order to protect the abandoned child in her: the child that had to be put into care by her mother, my other grandmother.

'You have, Mum. You really have.'

Nick's email comes into my head again – *'work out why you really want to do this'* – and I know that I'm doing it not just for the children I never had but also for all the children without the families they long for, children like my mum and dad.

'I've got one more question, Mum . . .'

One more word to make twenty-one.

The word she gives me is 'mother'.

The One-Week Wait

When I started this Channel challenge I had no idea how many parallels there were going to be with going through IVF. I'll never know whether I would have done it if I had known. There's the physical and mental toughness of the training – just like IVF. There are all the things about succeeding that are out of your control – just like IVF. And now I realise there is also 'the wait'.

In IVF it's called the Two-Week Wait – the fourteen days between having your eggs collected and taking a pregnancy test to see if your treatment has worked. After all the prodding and poking you've endured over the previous weeks and months, once your embryos are put back inside you, you're suddenly left on your own. Time seems interminable and you become hyper-aware of every twinge or lack of twinge in your body, oscillating between thinking it's a positive sign and then a negative sign. But there's nothing you can do to influence the result. All you can do is wait.

In Channel swimming it's the One-Week Wait. On Friday 21 August my tidal window opens and I have seven days in which to swim. I have hired a big house in Capel-le-Ferne, a village between Dover and Folkestone, in order to sit the time out with my family. The house is perched right on the edge of the cliffs, looking out to sea, and in the promotional publicity it says it's the nearest house in England to France.

We arrive on the Friday: me, my mum, my sister, my brother-in-law, my niece, my niece's partner and her two children. One person is missing. When we are looking round the house, ten-year-old Jada takes my hand and asks: 'Where's Peter?' I'm floored by the question, even though I must have known it would come. I tell her he's away working and she nods, but I think she knows there's something else. We both know there's something else. Four-year-old Aaliyah is more interested in the house itself. 'Is this a palace?' she asks me, and later, much to her tearful disappointment, I get given the best room in the palace, with a gold-rimmed rococo bed and floor-to-ceiling windows leading out to a balcony looking out to sea. It feels wrong to be occupying the master bedroom alone, but there is no arguing with my sister's insistence that I am the guest of honour this week. So I accept it gratefully and Aaliyah eventually does too.

Paul, my pilot, has two swimmers to take ahead of me, and things start well, with Swimmer Number One going out on the first day of the tide and making it. One down, one to go. The next day the weather looks set to change for the worse and, along with several other pilots, Paul decides to stay ashore. However, come the end of the day he regrets his decision because it holds out long enough for some other swimmers and their pilots to make it across. It just shows what a game of chicken this is. Come Sunday it's still one down and one to go and the weather is now unquestionably taking a bad turn.

The previous day, Saturday, I had brought my family down to the beach to introduce them to the Dover team and for what I had envisaged would be a quick dip. Freda gave me three hours. OK, it's not seven, but I still nearly cried. The one thing I had been looking forward to in the final weeks of training was tapering and in the week of my swim I wasn't expecting anything more than an hour. It was as if she already knew that I wasn't going anywhere anytime soon. On Sunday Freda gives me another three hours and at the end of it I'm exhausted, as much from the stress of being given it and fearing what it means as from actually doing it. There's a reason that people say the wait is one of the hardest parts of swimming the Channel. Just like the two-week period in IVF, the mental anguish of not knowing what the result will ultimately be is excruciating.

With our relay last year, it hadn't felt as bad. Like the first time you go through IVF, there was an innocence about the wait because I'd never done it before and didn't know what to expect. Then we were slot four of our tidal week, so we knew we wouldn't go at the beginning and eventually, swam on the penultimate day of the tide. Last year I hadn't really given the weather a second thought, but now I know what can go wrong and I'm terrified about risking it. I've become obsessed not with monitoring twinges in my body but with wind speeds, even the smallest change. Every morning I come down to the kitchen and, whilst my sister makes the tea, I check the forecast on Windguru (there's a website and app for everything nowadays). Each day is made up of a horizontal line of boxes spaced out at three-hour intervals, and each box has a number in it and is shaded in a different colour. Boxes with low numbers that are white or light blue are good; boxes with high numbers that are green, yellow and red are bad. Every few hours the site is updated and the numbers and colours shift. Sunday is green; Monday is green with a little bit of blue (but not enough). Tuesday is green with a little bit of yellow (i.e. worse than the day before). On the Tuesday Nick sends me an email with instructions for how to win at Monopoly. Like Freda, it's as if he knows the wait is going to continue. But there are only so many times you can buy Park Lane before you go crazy.

Wednesday is red – red is very bad. Thursday is yellow with a bit of green. Friday is green with an emerging bit of blue, but it doesn't matter now anyway: Friday is the last day of my tide and I haven't swum. No one has since last Saturday; the sea has been unswimmable. I've just endured a week of anxious anticipation in Capel-le-Ferne with my family for nothing. The next tide is a spring (the tide that's considered to be harder to swim than a neap) and the way it works is that the swimmers who are booked into the next tide go straight to the top of the queue. So not only have I had to sit through the wait of my own tidal week, I now have to keep waiting without any idea of when or if my swim will come at all.

I call Paul and he tells me that he's only got one swim booked on the next spring tide – a relay team from the military – and as the weather is finally improving he's decided to take them tomorrow, Saturday. He tells me if that things go well there could be a chance for Swimmer Number Two of my tidal week to go on Sunday and for me to follow him on Monday, if I'm prepared to brave the spring. Right now I feel like I'm prepared to brave anything rather than continue indefinitely into the unknown.

We have only rented our palace for the week and my family have to go home, so I book myself into the Premier Inn in order to stay on for the weekend, waiting, whilst they head back to London, promising to return if they get word that I'm going. As they wave me goodbye after a final lunch in the White Horse pub, the legendary hostelry where all successful Channel swimmers get to sign their name, Jada calls after me: 'Remember, Aunty Jessica, pain is temporary, glory is forever,' words she had read on the wall of the pub that had captured her ten-year-old imagination. Although the week hasn't been what I imagined, the wait has bonded us as a family in a deep and lasting way, and watching the girls swim in the shallows of the shore where Barrie feeds us, and swimming out to my favourite red bucket on the right with my sister, has been something to treasure, whatever happens next.

On Saturday I head to the beach. Freda gives me a two hour swim: could she be finally accepting my time is coming? Later that evening I call Paul again for an update. He sounds grumpy. He's still at sea with the soldier relayers, some of whom he says can hardly swim, but they're not giving up the fight. He won't be back until very late, which means if he does take Swimmer Number Two tomorrow he won't get any sleep. He's noncommittal about what his exact plans are. More uncertainty.

———————

Sunday dawns. A glorious day. I head to the beach and the team confirm that Paul and Swimmer Number Two have gone out this morning. Instead of feeling relieved that I'm now next in line, I feel intensely jealous. All I can think is that if Paul had made the decision to take Swimmer Two out on the Saturday of my tidal week – which in retrospect he should have done – today might have been my day. The conditions look perfect. Freda gives me another two hours.

After training, I ring Paul, who picks up my call at sea and tells me that Swimmer Number Two is making good progress and things are looking hopeful for me going tomorrow but to ring again after the 6 p.m. forecast. I spend the afternoon purchasing supplies for my support team. Coffee, tea, packet soups, pot noodles, cakes and biscuits, all the things they'll need for what could be twenty-four hours on a small boat at sea. At six I call again. Things are still looking possible for tomorrow and Paul tells me to get my support team on standby. I ring John to tell him but there is terrible news for me and for him. His elderly mother, who I knew was ill with cancer, has suddenly taken a turn for the worse and he can't leave her bedside. A highly stressful hour ensues, trying to find someone else to take over. I should be eating, sleeping or at least trying to sleep, but instead life has created another hurdle for me. At around 10 p.m., all my team members finally in place and some of them already on their way, I get into bed.

Then suddenly, out of nowhere – not even out of a little coloured box on Windguru – a jagged light cracks across the Channel and a huge storm erupts. Lightning illuminates the sky in the sort of firework display only nature can create. My first thought is not for me, but for Swimmer Number Two, who has now been at sea for over thirteen hours and is still out there. Rain starts lashing down and I just can't believe there's any way a swimmer could survive it.

I ring Freda in a frenzy, waking her up. She sounds cross and I feel awful, although she does assure me that it's very unlikely that a swimmer would be hit by lightening. But as the storm continues unabated, I can't believe that anyone could continue out there and within an hour news comes through that the swim has been aborted. And now all I can think is: it could have been me. If Paul, my pilot, had taken Swimmer Number Two last Saturday, like he should have done, then I would have swum today and round about now it would all have been over. It's like the two-week wait in IVF when the blood comes: there's no surer sign that Nature's made her decision.

Tomorrow's swim is off. I call my support team to tell them that standby is now stand-down. The following day is bank holiday Monday and I have been in Dover for a week and three days straight. I head to the beach: bank holidays are treated like weekends for training purposes and all the team are there, although the number of swimmers is now dwindling as tomorrow it's September and the end of the season is approaching. It's drizzling, which matches exactly how I feel. I apologise profusely to Freda for waking her up. She acts as if she's still cross but she's just teasing; she thanks me for giving her the opportunity to see such a magnificent firework display. And what's more, she doesn't even suggest that I should get into the water. Instead she, Barrie and Irene all tell me it's time to get out of Dover and go home. The One-Week Wait is over but the waiting continues. I head back to London, defeated.

Are You Asleep Yet?

I wake up on Tuesday morning. I know I've got to muster the energy to go in to work. A watched line of coloured boxes never changes. Besides, I can't stay away indefinitely, waiting for something I don't know will come. I pad into the kitchen to make myself a cup of tea and take it back to bed to drink before getting up properly. I open my laptop, automatically click on Windguru, as I have done every day for the last ten days, and to my astonishment the boxes for tomorrow have turned white. Well, a couple are light blue, but most of them are white. I stare at the screen in disbelief. Last night they were green. I'm sure they were green. Is white really white? I pick up my phone and text Paul: 'Are my eyes seeing what I think they're seeing?' I write. 'Could we go tomorrow?' Within a few minutes my phone rings and Paul concurs that it does look possible if we leave at midnight tonight, but he'll confirm after the noon forecast.

I ring work and tell my lovely PA that I won't come in, just in case, but not to tell anyone anything yet. The morning drags. I text Nick to see what he thinks but don't get a reply. I text Freda to ask the same. Again, I hear nothing. I pace the flat and count the minutes. At noon on the dot I check Windguru again: the boxes are still looking white. I want to call Paul but he's told me to wait until he calls me. At 12:16 I get a text from Nick: 'Tomorrow's forecast is a definite GO GO GO!' A few minutes later a text from Freda: 'God no sleep for me tonight.' But still no word from Paul. At 12:48 I can't contain myself and text him: 'It's looking good, isn't it? Should I go to bed this afternoon to sleep?' And within seconds my phone pings and Paul says: 'Are you asleep yet?'

The wait is over. I'm going. Tonight.

Dear Peter

Dear Peter,

I'm writing to let you know how it went. I always thought you'd be there, sharing every moment with me and consoling me when I failed, like you've done so many times before. But you weren't, so now words on a page must suffice. It's funny that today is the third of September – my mum and dad's wedding anniversary. I always remember my dad telling me when I was little that it was the day the war broke out, and then he'd chuckle at his double entendre. But for me today is a day of peace.

I've been thinking about the first time I told you I wanted to swim the Channel. I remember calling you from work. You were incredulous and asked why I'd never mentioned it before. But I reminded you it had been on my bucket list, those ones we did when we were away after another unsuccessful round of IVF. Top of my list was to become a mother; top of your list was for me to become a mother too. Swimming the Channel was my number nine – I know because I've still got those lists and I've checked. But you'd forgotten about them, and to be honest I'd forgotten about them too until they teased me at work about doing a sponsored swim.

After your initial incredulity, I remember you got cross. I know you'll say you weren't but you were. You said it was stupid to consider doing something so difficult and dangerous when I wasn't really a swimmer and I've always hated exercise and the cold. I can't remember who put down the phone first – was it me, or you? But gradually, over time, you realised I was serious, and then came your unswerving support, as you have always given me. Just like when you looked at me across the dinner table that Christmas and mouthed: 'Let's do it.'

You would drive me to the Serpentine before work, sit on a bench in the cold, concerned that I couldn't seem to swim in a straight line. But you also told me I looked good in the water – even though we both knew I was slow and most of the other swimmers in the lake overtook me. And I'll never forget when I did my first ever six hours in the Oasis, seeing your feet at the end of the pool.

But then there was Formentera. When I got out of the water after my qualifier everyone thought I was crying because I'd done it – me, the person who a year before had struggled to swim ten minutes in the same bay – but I was crying because you were supposed to be there and hadn't come. You weren't there for my first seven and six either, but when I was swimming across the harbour I let myself dream you might be waiting with a towel; I even thought I saw you standing on the beach, but it wasn't you. And you weren't there yesterday, on 2 September, when the wait was over and the day had finally come. You will always be the missing piece of this story. But that's what you wanted, wasn't it . . .

———————

We got to the harbour at around midnight, loaded everything onto the boat. The official observer – her name was Loretta – took me below deck to fill out the official forms. She asked me how I wanted my name to appear on my certificate and I immediately thought: 'If there is one.'

If: the smallest word in the English language with the biggest meaning, the one that Freda gave me.

We set off out of the harbour. Paul told me not to start getting ready until fifteen minutes before we reached Samphire Hoe. Someone said I looked calm and I did feel more relaxed than I thought I would when this moment finally came. Maybe it was the relief that the wait had finished, that whatever happened now it would all be over soon. When we were getting near, I went up on deck. I already had my costume on underneath my clothes – my favourite blue one with the red and white stripes – so it didn't take long to get ready. I put on my red hat with Webb's words – 'nothing great is easy' – emblazoned on it: I needed those with me. As I got undressed, the team held me steady on the rocking boat and covered me all over with suncream and Vaseline. I said I felt like the Queen of Sheba. (In fact, who was the Queen of Sheba? Was she a mother?)

The boat slowed and then it stopped. I couldn't see the shore; all about us was black. And then everything happened so quickly; there was no messing around. I climbed down the steps at the back of the boat into the water, everyone's eyes on me. This was the bit I had been dreading; just the thought of it made my heart skitter. But when it finally came I actually felt surprisingly composed. Maybe it was the darkness, which made it difficult to see my fear. Or maybe it was because fear is always worse in your imagination. Like the fear of not becoming a mother. I wonder now, after everything I've learned from the women I've met, if the thought of not being a mother is worse than it will actually be.

I had already warned everyone that I would be breaststroking the hundred or so metres to shore to reach the start point – my small concession to comfort before an Everest of crawl. Before I got out of the water, I carefully adjusted my goggles, licking the inside of the lenses, dipping them and putting them on again, tightening the strap. I stumbled on the pebbles in the dark, then turned, stood for a moment and raised my arms above my head. There was a second's hesitation, when I wasn't sure whether they could see me on the boat. There wasn't the claxon I was expecting, but the lights on the boat flashed and I knew it was time to go. I checked my watch: 1:30 a.m. I stepped forward. I was in.

The first hour was fine. I enjoyed the darkness, the warmth of the water against the cold night air, the sound of the boat putting along beside me. Five minutes before my feed the team twirled a light stick, as they'd said they would. And then five minutes later they twirled two to indicate it was time. I moved closer to the boat. Someone shouted something I couldn't hear. They dropped the feed bottle on a line into the water. I drank it without a word and continued. They'll be pleased with that, I thought: I'd fed quickly and hadn't stopped to chat or complain. I felt focused and had nothing to complain about – yet.

Hour two was good. One twirling light, then two five minutes later. But things were about to change. At hour three, I couldn't face my feed and I asked for water instead. I was starting to feel nauseous, it was creeping through my insides, but I didn't want anyone to know. I swam on. The first time I vomited, I managed it quietly into the swell. But then I started to feel worse. Soon I couldn't hide it and every few strokes I stopped, violently retching into the sea, sounding just as Nick had said: like an animal in pain. I don't know what made me sick. Was it nerves? I didn't think it was nerves; I'd felt so calm at the start. Was it the fumes from the boat? Was it the fact that it was one of the first times I'd taken feed that I'd made myself, and it was stronger and more frequent than I was used to having in training? What I do know is this. When I started to feel ill, really ill, I realised that Boris was right when he'd told me that however hard you trained the real thing was going to be a magnitude bigger.

Boris was on the boat – he had agreed to take over from John as captain of my support team. I didn't want to let him down after all the advice he'd given me, but I started to fear

I couldn't do it: a sinking feeling that despite all my training, none of it had been enough. Then to my right, suddenly in the darkness, loomed a mass of twinkling lights. In each short moment as my face turned out of the water to breathe I tried to work out what it was. In my delirium I couldn't comprehend it: it looked like a palace in the sea, big and beautiful and strange. I realise now it must have been a cruise ship passing in the night, but I was bewildered by it and vomited again.

Five minutes before hour four they gave me my warning, and then everyone disappeared inside the boat. I swam on, wondering what was happening, convinced that five minutes had passed and that I should be being fed. Not that I wanted food, but I wanted the company of people on the deck. When I turned and breathed to my left I could see a group of shadowy figures in the cabin talking. I had no idea what was going on. I learned later they were trying to work out what to do. Paul was cross at how little progress I was making. The tide and my slow speed in it was taking me horizontally along the Dover cliffs and not across to France. And my support team were discussing what they could possibly feed me that had any chance of staying down. Sickness was a challenge, but sickness without replacement sustenance would surely be terminal. Eventually, they came out on deck and called me over and gave me a cup of hot chocolate. I vomited it back up and swam on. Then Paul leaned out of the captain's window and gave me a pot of porridge. As I grabbed it, I dunked it into the sea, ate one salty mouthful, handed it back and was sick again. But the worst thing of all they gave me in those horrendous next few hours was strong, sweetened black tea. Or maybe it was the best thing, because it made me so sick that after that I wasn't sick again.

As daylight broke I tried my best to lift my spirits. I had been longing for the light. It was a beautiful morning and the sunrise was stunning, but it was difficult to appreciate it because the pain and exhaustion was so intense. But things were about to change again, this time for the better, and bizarrely my salvation would be my nemesis: jellyfish.

The first sting was on my arm and to be honest it wasn't wholly unpleasant. It was like brushing a nettle, and after the sickness this new sensation gave me something else to think about. The second sting was across my face and that was a shock. And after that they kept on coming, their formless bodies floating into my path. We seemed unable to avoid each other. At my next feed I shouted upwards, 'Bloody jellyfish,' because I wasn't sure whether they could see them on the boat. Everyone on deck nodded. They could see them. Soon there wasn't just the odd one, like in our jellyfish film at home, moving elegantly across the screen as they pulsed slowly in and out to their jellyfish music. No, soon I was swimming through jellyfish soup. They were everywhere, at times thick like oil slicks. And there were all different kinds; the worst ones had long tendrils which one of them wrapped round my arm, making me yelp with pain. This went on for several hours, sometimes with a short respite, maybe because of a clump of seaweed which soothed the throbbing, but then they'd be back again.

But, as I said, the bizarre thing was the jellyfish were in

fact my saviours. My stroke rate increased, probably because I was trying to get away from them. And the fact is that once you've been stung a hundred times you stop feeling the pain. So as I swam into another smack, I simply said, 'Hi, Mr Jellyfish, nice to see you again.'

During the jellyfish hours something had shifted. The tide had turned and I had covered a lot of distance. I didn't know it at first but then I noticed Loretta, the observer, was standing on deck watching me and every now and then, when my head turned towards her, she would clap. And then Paul leaned out of the captain's cabin and gave me a thumbs-up. I didn't understand what was happening but I thought it must be a good sign. My support team were there to encourage me, and their words of motivation and praise at every feed couldn't necessarily be trusted. When Boris told me I was about halfway, I didn't actually believe him. But I figured Loretta and Paul had no vested interest in me succeeding. In fact, if I wasn't going to make it, the sooner I got out, the sooner they could get back to England. So when they clapped and gave me the thumbs-up that was something to pay heed to.

I swam on, encouraged. And yet the worst part was still to come.

Cap Gris-Nez. I'd heard those three words so many times – the nearest point in France from England and where the fastest swimmers land. Slower swimmers generally come in further down the coast towards Calais, so I never imagined for a moment that I would see it, but suddenly there it was: a cylindrical lighthouse on the cliff rising up ahead of me. At first, I couldn't quite believe it. Like the palace in the sea I'd seen during the night, it felt like another mirage. But now it was daylight and the coast of France was clearly visible ahead. I was sure it was Cap Gris-Nez.

I was right – that wasn't my mistake. My mistake was thinking that it wasn't far and all I had to do was swim towards it in a straight line. Rejuvenated by the sight, I swam on. For the first time I felt there was a chance I could do it. I even allowed myself to look at my watch and spent a good while trying to work out how long I had been in the water. In my tiredness, I found it difficult to count, unable to connect the time I started with the number of hours between then and now, but eventually I estimated I had been swimming for around thirteen hours, and reckoned, from the land ahead, I had about another two to go. I couldn't believe it. Me – me! Could I make it to France in fifteen hours? No wonder Loretta and Paul were pleased after the slow start.

Maybe it was while I was distracted by all this that Cap Gris-Nez disappeared. Suddenly the French coast looked further than it had before and I was swimming alongside it, not towards it.

At my next feed, Boris congratulated me and said I had finally reached French waters. I think this was supposed to encourage me but in fact I felt deflated. Given the proximity of France, or so it seemed from the water, I had genuinely thought I was nearly there. But I wasn't. What had happened was the tide had turned again and was taking me along the coast towards Calais, and what I hadn't realised was that once the tide turns there is no way of breaking it until it slacks and lets you through; I just had to swim. And despite the sickness, the jellyfish, the hours I had already swum, this was about to be by far the worst bit because, regardless of all I had learned about the Channel, I didn't understand what had happened and I had no idea how long it would go on. When I saw Cap Gris-Nez I had allowed myself to do something fatal. I had relaxed a little, like you do in the last ten minutes of a swim, when you know you'll soon be able to get out. Even then you've still got to swim a terrible ten minutes, but now the ten minutes really was going to be hours.

Mentally, I knew something in me was starting to give up. At the next feed, I abandoned all promise not to complain and shouted: 'It's not getting any closer.' At every feed thereafter I repeated this desperate mantra. 'It *is*,' they'd shout from the boat, but I didn't believe them. I could see what I could see. The land ahead ebbed and flowed but overall it wasn't getting any nearer to me. And then I asked the question you're never supposed to ask: 'How long have I got?'

Paul leaned out of the boat and shouted: 'You've got as long as it takes to get there.'

Up until now I realised I had thought very little during the swim. My consciousness had been punctuated by sickness, stings, the dark, the light, cruise ships and Lego-like tankers crossing the separation zone, but I hadn't actually thought of anything. All I had done was swim. Now I needed something desperately and, for the first time since I'd got in the sea, I summoned the words of the women I'd met. With each stroke, as I slapped my arm down on the water, I went through my list of twenty-one words:

Arigatou-gozaimasu. Slap.

Can. Slap.

Courage. Slap, breathe.

Delicious. Slap.

Determination. Slap.

Doggedness. Slap, breathe.

Eschatological. Slap.

Grit. Slap.

If. Slap, breathe.

Keep Going. Slap.

Life. Slap.

Mother. Slap, breathe.

Mystery. Slap.

Om. Slap.

Opportunity. Slap, breathe.

Ozymandias. Slap.

Persistence. Slap.

Privilege. Slap, breathe.

Ruth. Slap.

Strength. Slap.

Water. Slap, breathe.

When I reached the word 'water', I thought about all the hours I'd spent in it over the last two years and that, however long this swim was, it was just a day, just one day in my life, and nothing compared to what I'd already swum to get here. And that if I could keep going on this one day then I'd never have to swim seven and six in the harbour again. In fact, I'd never have to swim again at all. But if I didn't keep going then, like all the times I failed at IVF, something in me would make me do it all over again – because I'm not good at giving up. I realise that now. And then I thought about the last words that Jada had shouted after me when my family left me in Dover: 'Remember, Aunty Jessica, pain is temporary, glory is forever.'

Pain-is-temporary. Slap. Glory-is-forever. Slap.

This time my ten minutes really did last for five hours. Suddenly there was movement at the back of the boat and Boris was climbing down the steps into the water beside me. Boris, who had been at the Serpentine the first time I went on that cold, wet Saturday morning. Boris, who had written to me a year ago and said I had to hurt myself every day from now on, because he knew. Boris, who had been my doubter, but who, like so many of my new-found Channel-swimming family, had also remained true. He started swimming one-armed crawl. He was still faster than me. And then he said: 'Just one more length to the end of the Serpentine.'

I heard him almost unbelievingly. 'Just one more length and then you're there. Then, Jessica, you'll be a Channel swimmer.'

It was only when my feet brushed the bottom that I believed I had actually made it. I let one leg reach down. Then two legs, and the seabed was under my feet. I felt the rush of water around me and, wobbling and unsteady, I moved forward. The beach ahead looked beautiful: white sand, the sun just starting to set. I said later it looked like the Maldives and everyone laughed and said that Sangatte wasn't quite as beautiful as that. But it was to me. It was my Maldives. I cleared the water and turned so they could see me back on the boat. The sand was soft, the beach was wide and empty. And I had always thought that if this moment ever came I would jump and shout and punch the air, but in fact I just held my hands to my chest and, shivering slightly, looking back out to sea, I murmured: 'I did it. I swam from England to France. I did it.'

Seventeen hours, forty-four minutes and thirty seconds of labour, followed by the most extraordinary euphoria that immediately eclipsed all the pain. I'd done something big and life would never be the same again. And when I'd collected my pebble (which was actually a mussel shell because there were no pebbles around); and when I'd swum back to the boat (well, Boris swam, he gave me a lift on his back); and after the team had helped me change and gasped at the jellyfish stings which were all over my arms and legs, and then given me a cup of hot water because that's all I could face, I was just happy to be with people and in the warmth of the boat; the first thing I said after all this, as the realisation that I had actually done it started to finally sink in, was: 'Does Peter know? Does Peter know I made it?'

The Last Supper

I may never be able to say that I was the 4 million and 91st woman to give birth to an IVF baby, but I will always be able to say that I was the 491st woman to swim the English Channel. There may never be answerphone messages or cards of congratulations on the birth of a baby girl or boy, but there will always be the hundreds of messages I received for what I did that day in the sea, which in a strange way felt like I was giving birth to me.

It's true, like John said at the start: I don't want to eat much for a week, and ten stone seems like a distinct possibility for a while. But becoming a Channel swimmer, well, that is cause for celebration, and there was one more question I'd asked each of the women I'd met: what would be their last supper? Eating their choices was to be my reward. And after a week, I am ready to feast.

I decide to get the healthy stuff out of the way first – that means fruit. I have to say that if I was sitting down with Jesus or heading for the chair, fruit wouldn't be my first choice. But for three of my women it was. Businesswoman Nicola Horlick told me she doesn't really like eating and if she could simply have fruit for every meal she would. She said she wanted mangoes, pawpaws, passion fruit, strawberries, raspberries and peaches. Somehow it feels wrong to me to buy them in a supermarket. If it has to be fruit, I want romance. So I decide to make a special trip to Andreas in Chelsea, the oft-crowned grocer of the year.

I choose the peaches not just for Nicola but also for Diana Athill, the publisher and writer. I had wanted to meet a woman at the end of her life who hadn't had children to see how it felt facing old age and death without descendants around you. Although she didn't agree to meet me she did answer three questions I put to her in an email, each with one word: 1) Do you regret not having children? *No.* 2) Could you give me a word for my swim? *Courage.* And 3) What would be your last supper? *Peaches.*

I remember how Gertrude Ederle had eaten a peach before her swim and it had made her feel sick. I will never know what made me so sick in the sea, but now that I'm out, it's double peaches for me.

Kim Longinotto, my filmmaker, chose mangoes and when she did we had the 'how do you eat a mango?' conversation because it is definitely a fruit that requires some practice to master. The only way to eat it with relative dignity is to slice it down each side, avoiding the core, and then score the flesh with a knife in a grid and turn the skin down and out. (Maybe it was because I reminded Kim of the complications of eating a mango that she changed her mind and chose a piece of dry Ryvita instead. She said that actually if it was her last supper she wouldn't want to regret the joys of life.) But the joys of life should be celebrated so I take my prizes home and make myself a huge fruit salad, for Nicola, Diana and Kim.

From fruit, I progress to sushi, which would also not be my first last choice. Two women had chosen it: my anonymous mother and Justine Roberts of Mumsnet. Justine recommended I go to a restaurant called Tajima-Tei in Leather Lane, which she said served the best sushi in London. I like a woman who recommends restaurants, even if it's just for raw fish, so I go to eat their house sushi and drink ice-cold sake from a box. It's delicious. From sushi, I move on to Asian fusion, as my macrobiotic mother, Claudia Spahr, had chosen buckwheat noodles and tempeh with ginger and soya sauce.

Like sushi and sake, jacket potatoes also featured twice. My ballerina, Deborah Bull, wanted houmous on one half and cheese on the other, with an avocado and bean-sprout salad (because, she said, they crush down nicely). My general, Freda Streeter, just wanted one with cheese. I remember how Freda cried when I asked her this question and said that two years ago, before her husband died, she would have chosen pasta because they loved eating lasagne together, but there just wasn't any point in cooking any more. I resolve that I must ring her and go round, feed the fish, watch the tree and make her lasagne. She says that she's retiring this year but no one believes her. Maybe no one wants to believe her because Dover beach wouldn't be the same without Freda.

After fruit, sushi and jacket potatoes, I decide to travel to

Persia – well, Persian London – for Camila Batmanghelidjh's dish of choice. She was another woman who professed to not like food very much and said her last supper would be a plate of sour spinach from the Galleria restaurant in Marylebone.

Jackie Cobell, Ice Queen Foster Mother, simply wanted crusty bread and butter. She said it was the thing she most craved when her jaws were wired up in one of her many bids to lose weight before she embarked on her record-breaking journey to swim the Channel. I asked whether she wanted the butter to be salted or unsalted. 'Salted, I think,' she replied. Personally, I wouldn't have had to think about it. Butter on bread just has to be salted for me. It's the one thing I definitely share with the sea.

Fiona Shackleton, my divorce lawyer, wanted an omelette. Plain or possibly with *fines herbes* and most definitely *baveuse*, she said. I had to look up *baveuse* because, although I may have swum to France, my French isn't very good. Thankfully, she wasn't suggesting I ate it with a baby's bib (that's *bavoir*); an *omelette baveuse* has to be soft and runny, folded over in a half-circle of sun. She wanted it with a tomato and onion salad, heavy balsamic vinegar and nice bread.

For my chief constable's last supper I have to wait until a Sunday. Julie Spence wanted roast dinner and that's the day of the week it tastes best. She's a vegetarian, remember so she wanted roast beef and Yorkshire pudding without the roast beef. I did have to protest a bit. The thought of roast dinner without the meat just doesn't feel right. She also wanted water with it and not wine. A Sunday roast without a glass of red is another anathema to me. But she's the chief constable and I wasn't about to get another lunch wrong. So I have her preferred glass of water (followed by an Americano with hot milk).

My recompense is that I can follow Julie's alcohol-free, vegetarian roast lunch later in the week with steak, because two women had ordered it. The first was my Gateway Woman, Jody Day. She wanted sirloin steak, frites and a green salad with a glass of Pinot Noir. The polar explorer, Ann Daniels, also wanted steak because, she said, it's the antidote to slop. But even more importantly, she wanted to eat her last supper sitting at a table on a chair. Her answer had taken her back to the Arctic, when all her meals were runny and had to be eaten hunched in her tent. I hadn't asked Ann's daughter, Sarah, what she wanted. But I eat chips for her. All children like chips. Don't they?

There was only one woman who chose just something sweet – my Ironwoman Eddie Brocklesby, who said she'd have a blackcurrant ice lolly. But what was fascinating about her answer was that my question didn't make her think about what her favourite food was. It made her think about death and how when you're dying it can be very difficult to swallow, so what you want is something you can taste and don't have to chew. She said that maybe her answer was because over her life she'd seen one or two deaths too many including, of course, her husband's. It made me think about how grief made me swim and her run.

Then there were the women who wanted three courses,

the women after my own heart and stomach. My politician Fiona Mactaggart knew what she wanted immediately. She'd obviously thought about the subject before. Scallops, black pudding and pea shoots with balsamic vinegar glaze, followed by Dover sole, asparagus and new potatoes, and then raspberries with Greek yoghurt for dessert. All this was to be accompanied by a bottle of Clos des Mouches. My Very Reverend Lorna Hood wanted almost exactly the same starter – scallops, black pudding and pea puree (rather than shoots). I eat them on consecutive days to economise my purchases. Lorna also wanted fish for her main, but for her it was halibut with cauliflower cheese and creamy mashed potato, followed by sticky toffee pudding. I forgot to ask her about a drink so I finish off Fiona's Clos des Mouches.

My scientist, Susan Greenfield, was very clear about her drink: she wanted pink champagne. And then for starters garlicky snails with French baguette and butter. I have to say I'm not a massive fan of snails. I wish I were, but we had a house once with a garden that was rife with them. I can't face cooking them at home so I decide to go to Mon Plaisir, one of the oldest French restaurants in London. For her main, Susan wanted liver with creamy mashed potato and onions. I know that many people are as squeamish about liver as they are about snails, but thankfully, I'm not one of them. I love it. My only disappointment was that she didn't add some spinach on the side, so I make that executive decision for her. And to finish she didn't want a pudding but runny camembert. There's nothing better than finishing a delicious meal with cheese, although strictly speaking if you're going for the works – which I am – you need a pudding and *then* cheese, so I make another amendment and have a lemon tart first. Apologies to the French, who allowed me onto their soil without going through border control, for not preferring it the other way around, but I'm definitely English where pudding and cheese is concerned.

And so to my cook and restaurateur.

'What would be your last supper?' I asked Prue Leith.

'How many courses?' she piercingly enquired.

'That's for you to decide, but I can eat a lot of courses, so don't worry about me.'

'Well, we've been talking about cassoulet and motherly things and I think I'd probably have—' she breaks her train of thought to say that somebody else has probably already chosen it and she'll back off if they have, and then continues on track '—but I think I'd like really good sausages and onion gravy and mash.'

I told her it was fine, she could have them, as she was the first.

'And would you prefer to have it at home or out?' I asked.

'For my last meal? I think I'd have it at home.'

Home and family and sausage and mash. What could be more perfect?

'I absolutely love picnics too,' she continued, as if the sausages were suddenly not enough. 'I like ones that are very old-fashioned. A hard-boiled egg in a piece of paper – a gull's egg rather than hen's – with celery salt to dip it in. And then sandwiches on really good bread, thin with the crusts cut off and lots of filling. Smoked salmon sandwiches with really good salmon, and avocado sandwiches with a bit of chilli. And then Eton mess – meringue, cream and strawberries in little plastic yoghurt pots. And lots of champagne, of course.'

Prue told me how they would have this picnic every year on the fourth of June at her son's school – Eton. They would take a rug down to the Thames and watch the boys rowing. Some of the other families would have their picnics out of the back of their Range Rovers and to Prue's embarrassment some people even had their picnics catered by her own company, but for Prue, a picnic has to be homemade, sitting on a rug on the ground. That could be her last lunch, she said.

'And then home for sausages and mash in the evening?' I suggested.

'Yes, exactly. That's fine. That will do me.'

It would do me too. There was nothing about Prue's description that was a touchstone of my own childhood but it was a perfect image of the one I had longed to create. And then I thought of my mum and how when I asked her the question she had simply said, 'with the family'; she didn't care what the food was. So after my swim in the Indian summer of September, I created Prue's last supper for Mum – a picnic and a walk on Hampstead Heath – we remembered my dad. And then home for sausages and mash. Because although neither of us ever quite had the family of our dreams, we do have the family of our reality and that will always be something to treasure.

Epilogue

'Seven-hour lamb?'

'Why not!'

'Potatoes?'

'Better not. I'm not in training any more.'

'That never stopped you before.'

I smile.

It's two months after my swim; nearly Christmas again. A lot has happened. I've left my job, turned forty-five and am about to leave for Africa to climb Kilimanjaro with fourteen strangers. I booked it all in a blur soon after the swim. The comedown after the climax was bigger than I expected. When I rang Freda the next morning, before she'd even said congratulations, she warned: 'Now listen to me, mate, you're going to get depressed. It's normal.'

She was right – I had got my happy ending, but life is not a book. It goes on. There's always an epilogue. As the end of the year approaches, I'm not just dreading Christmas without children any more, I'm now dreading Christmas without the Channel, as well as the prospect that I might be spending it without Peter. Over the last few months we have been living increasingly separate lives. He's been sleeping I'm not sure where, and I've been sleeping alone at our flat. We've been talking by text because when we do talk we fall out. But we've arranged to meet up for supper before I leave for Africa.

'I never thought you wouldn't be there,' I say.

'I wanted to be there.'

'I wanted that too. More than anything.'

'No you didn't,' he contradicts me.

'Yes I did. But that's the problem, we each have our truth.'

A moment's silence settles between us and we both take a sip of Negroni.

'So did you get the answer to your question?' he asks.

'What question?'

'Whether motherhood makes you happy?'

'Yes.'

He looks at me as if he's waiting for me to continue.

'Yes,' I say again. 'The answer to the question is yes.'

'Oh,' he seems surprised and a bit crestfallen, as if he hoped I was going to say something different.

Our starter arrives. Crab on toast. Peter immediately discards the bread.

'But it's OK,' I continue. 'I also learned there are many ways to become a mother if you really want to. It's just that sometimes you have to adjust the route to get there.'

'Well, you definitely know about going off route. For a

while you weren't swimming to France, you were heading to Holland,' he says.

I laugh. 'Yeah, six hours in and they didn't think I stood a chance.'

'But you turned it around. You did something big.'

The waiter comes over to take our plates.

'Did you make a final decision on the potatoes?' he asks.

Peter looks at me.

'I think we'll be fine with just the lamb,' I say.

The waiter nods and Peter smiles. But it's a sad smile. Almost as if he's disappointed.

'So in the end doing something big wasn't enough?' he asks.

'Oh, it was. I wouldn't change it for anything.'

'Not even a baby?'

'Not even our baby.'

'But I thought you've found out that it's motherhood that makes you happy.'

'Yeah, but that's not all I learned. I learned that most people need something else in their life as well. Motherhood can make you happy, but it's rarely enough.'

I fill our glasses with Douro as the lamb arrives on a large oval plate; after seven hours in the oven it's falling off the bone and beautifully tender. As I serve us both I think that what I have learned over the last two years is that one of the reasons being a mother is so important is because humans are happiest when they have connection with other people. Parenthood is often the quickest route to that connection but it doesn't always work and it doesn't mean that you can't create the connection in other ways, with other members of your family (up, down and across). Or with your husband, wife or partner. Or with friends, especially those who have been in your life for a long time. You can even make extraordinary connections with strangers who you meet and (sometimes) eat with. Or with whole communities of strangers, like those who think that swimming in the open water is the bee's knees, the cat's whiskers and even the duck's poo. Connection is vital to human happiness, and if you can't get it ready-made by having your own children you need to create it in different ways.

But there's also something else I've learned, and that is that people are most fulfilled when they have a passion. Sometimes your children can be that passion but many people need something else as well. It might be ballet dancing, making films, running your own business or saving lives. It might be going in search of wildlife around the world, skiing to the North Pole or completing Ironman competitions. It might even be swimming the English Channel. But you've got to find your passion in life because, along with connection, that's where true happiness lies.

'Do you know what the biggest thing I learned is?' I say after taking a long sip of wine.

'Tell me,' Peter says.

'The biggest thing I learned is that everyone has sad things in their life. Ours was not being able to make a baby. But every single person in this restaurant is dealing with something that hurts. Maybe like us they want a child, or they've lost one. Or they've lost someone else too early – a husband, a wife, a brother, a sister, a mother, a father, a friend. Or maybe they don't feel like they've reached their potential or that anyone truly cares about them, or maybe—' I take another sip and look at him, '—the person they thought was their soulmate suddenly disappeared. But every single person in the world seems to have something that makes them terribly sad. And life is about making the best of your sad thing. That's why the Channel was enough, because it made the best of mine.'

'That's beautiful,' Peter says.

'Is it? It's a shame, really, that we're fundamentally all sad and that life is about making up for that. But I think it's true.'

'Is that why you're going to climb Kilimanjaro for Christmas?'

'Yeah, and I want to be up high near to the sky and the sun after all those months looking down into the cold dark sea.'

'I wish I was coming with you.'

'I wish you were too.'

He puts down his fork and pushes his plate aside. I pour the last of the Douro into both our glasses.

'Shall we have pudding?' he says.

'Pudding? You?'

'Why not.'

'Wow. OK. I'm not going to say no to that,' my voice quickens. 'I've already noticed they've got brown bread ice cream on the menu. Why don't I have a scoop of that and you have a scoop of the blood orange sorbet and we share?'

The ice cream arrives. The restaurant serves it in the same small glasses as they serve the Negronis, squashed in and leaning over the rim. They are the biggest two portions of ice cream you could hope for and we aren't able to finish them.

'I told you one scoop would be enough,' Peter says.

'You did.'

We both look down at the ice cream, defeated.

'Peter?'

'Yes.'

'If I asked you to give me a word for my Channel swim, just one word, what would it be?'

'But you don't need a word now. You've done it.'

'I know, but just imagine.'

He looks at me and without another beat, he says: 'The word I gave you was "love".'

Notes

Prologue

1 'The problem is,' I continue, 'I'm not sure anyone would vote in an "infertile" to run the country. Not when babies are what win elections.' In July 2016, Theresa May became the UK's prime minister following the resignation of David Cameron. May is childless. She has said that she and her husband wanted children but couldn't have them. Ironically, her appointment was aided by comments about her childlessness made by her rival in the Conservative Party leadership campaign, Andrea Leadsom – a mother of three. Leadsom said: 'I am sure Theresa will be really sad she doesn't have children so I don't want this to be "Andrea has children, Theresa hasn't" because I think that would be really horrible, but genuinely I feel that being a mum means you have a very real stake in the future of our country, a tangible stake.' There was a considerable backlash against these comments. Leadsom apologised to Theresa May 'for any hurt' she had caused, and withdrew from the leadership campaign shortly after.

['Andrea Leadsom Apologises to Theresa May over Motherhood Comments Row', *Independent*, 11 July 2016.]

Jessica Hepburn writes: thankfully, my prophecy was proved wrong but perhaps the furore proved my point.

The Charity Worker

2 a year after we meet it would close down In the summer of 2015, Kids Company went into receivership and was closed down amid widespread criticism of the leadership and governance of the charity.

Jessica Hepburn writes: I do not feel I know enough about the facts to comment on what happened at the charity. But I do believe that Camila Batmanghelidjh was wholly and genuinely committed to the children she was trying to help and that's why she maintains her very important place in my story.

The General

3 Queen of the Channel, Member of the Most Excellent Order of the British Empire (MBE) In the 2018 New Year Honours list Freda Streeter was also awarded an MBE for Services to Open-Water Swimming.

Jessica Hepburn writes: and that's karma too.

Acknowledgements

There are so many people I want to thank for *21 Miles*.

First the open-water swimming community. John and Alice (and all the amazing SwimQuest people I met along the way, including Catherine, Chris, Andy, Mark, Teresa). The Dover Beach Team (Freda, Barrie, Irene and Emma). Marcus from Durley. Nick and Sakura (for so much, including Camp Eton – and thanks again to Jeremy for being my swimming companion there). Deidre and Mike (you know you want to). The marvellous Ladies of the Lake – Eliza, Jan, Jaana, Kirstie, Mary and Nicola. In fact, everyone at the Serpentine. John and all who brave Wednesday nights at Charing Cross pool. My 'catch' coach Ray. My physio angel Alan. Ice Queen Jackie for her inspiration, but also Dave. The Channel Class of 2015, especially Kerry, Lisa, Volker and everyone whose coat-tails I swam on. Steve and Dom my relay buddies, and Tara for supporting us that day. And last, but never least, to my unparalleled Channel support team: Boris, Charlotte, Katie, Lyndel and Rod, plus Paul my pilot and Loretta, my observer. I would never have become a

Channel Swimmer without all of you – and you've changed my life for ever.

I must also thank all the wonderful women who agreed to be interviewed. I'm so grateful for your wisdom and it was a privilege to meet and (sometimes) eat with you.

And to everyone who has helped me turn twenty-one miles of sea into twenty-one miles of book. Peter for allowing me to tell our story (again) and without whose love I may never have become a writer. My agent Emily for her belief and support. Anna and Claire at New Writing North, who also believed and were instrumental. To the Unbound team (John, Kwaku, Jimmy, Imogen, Amy; and to Kate and Miranda for their brilliant editing and Katie for her film). Janet for agreeing to chair my first (and now second) book launch. And, of course, to everyone who pledged to make it happen. Bless you all.

Finally, there are just a few special people without whom my life over the last few years wouldn't have been as happy. Some of them appear in the pages of this book but all of them are an important part of the story. Cynthia, Joanne, Jada, Aaliyah, Beth, Tara, Vicky, Lyndel, Tracey, Ella, Katie, Gabby and my mum. Thank you girls for being the best of family and friends.

Patrons

Special thanks to these very important people and organisations who made a patron donation to *21 Miles*, and who believe in the power of the arts to change the world of fertility.

Fertility Fest – the world's first arts festival dedicated to fertility, infertility, modern families and the science of making babies which is supported by Arts Council England, Wellcome Trust, British Fertility Society and a consortium of forward-thinking fertility clinics including The Centre for Reproductive & Genetic Health (CRGH); Create Fertility; Fertility Plus; Gennet City Fertility; Lister Fertility Clinic; and London Women's Clinic.

Roger de Freitas
Liz Elston Mayhew
HammersmithLondon – with thanks also to Arun Sondhi and Patricia Bench
Louise Hepburn
Kate and Kevin McGrath
Caroline and Sandy Orr

Unbound is the world's first crowdfunding publisher, established in 2011.

We believe that wonderful things can happen when you clear a path for people who share a passion. That's why we've built a platform that brings together readers and authors to crowdfund books they believe in – and give fresh ideas that don't fit the traditional mould the chance they deserve.

This book is in your hands because readers made it possible. Everyone who pledged their support is listed below. Join them by visiting unbound.com and supporting a book today.

Sarah Acott

Ann Aitken

Judith Alexander

Sian Alexander

Emily Andreas

Alison Andrews

Vicky Arlidge

Caroline Armstrong

Dee Armstrong

Melissa Asare

Elizabeth (Liz) Ascham

Cathy Astley

Naomi Baird

Mette and Jon Barker

Katie Barlow

Sandra Bateman

Beth Beamer

James Beck

David Beidas

Kristen Bennett

Charlotte Benton

Katie Berlyn Holmes

Sarah Bloomfield

Katrina Bogan

Jacky Boivin

Anne Bonnar

Saskia Boujo

Carolyn Braby

Kate Brian

Samantha Brick

Tessa Broad

Kat Brown

David Brownlee

Nathan Bryon

Anna Burel

Ruth Butterworth

Rhiannon Cackett

Mary Cameron

Gayle Campbell

Lyn Carpenter

Mary Caws

Diane Chandler

Hazel Chapman www.
    courage2lead.com

Ed Chard

Sally Cheshire

Alix Clarke

Sheila Clarke

Adam Coleman

Harriet Combes

Rachel Congdon

Lesley Cook

Rosanna Cooper

Polly Courtney

Caroline Crewe-Read

Julia Croyden

Charlotte Cunningham

Emma Cunniffe

Chris Curry

Kelly Da Silva

Marilyn Daish

Mike Davidson and
    Liz Williamson

Kim Davies

Isabel Davis

Russell Davis

Jody Day

Roger de Freitas

Hannah Dell

Jasmine Dellal

Sian Dibben

Anna Disley

Belinda Donovan – in memory
    of Celia Mosely

Joanna Down

Felicity Duarte

Sarah Duguid

Anne Dunford

Stephen Dunn

Natasha Dyer

Shantel Ehrenberg

Arabella El Barkouki

Janet Ellis

Liz Elston Mayhew

Ana Maria Ene

Gillian Evans

Mark Faure Walker

Fertility Network UK

Megumi Fieldsend

Jaki Fischel-Bock

Sarah Floud

Andrew Foster

Sarah Franklin

Sissy Gasson

Roddy Gauld

Bilyana Gencheva

Anna German

Jemima Gibbons

Rachel Giles

Anthi Glymidou

Caroline Goldsmith

Jenni Grainger

Kim M Grant

Stewart Grant

Elina Grigoriou

Zeynep Gurtin

Laura Hall

Clare Hall-Craggs

HammersmithLondon

Joanne Harper

Cat Harrison

Lyndel Harrison

Henrietta Harwood-Smith

Lynn (the fin) Hawkins

Rachel Haworth

Steve Hayes

Sarah Hensby

Louise Hepburn

Usha Junge Hepburn

Natalie Highwood

Peter Holland

Sean Holmes

Charlotte Hughes

Carol Hulley

Marion Hume

Juliet Humphries

A Hurst

Elizabeth Hurst

Leyla Hutchings

Vanessa Impey

Jo Ind

Sophie Ingleby

Sharon Jackson

Rebecca James

Ester Janko Mulcahy

Ella Jenkins

Catrin John

Ange Johnson

Lucy Johnson

Matthew Johnston

Alice Jolly

Jo Jones

Eliza Kaczynska-Nay

Kirendip Kandola

Pippa Kassam

Thomas Keen

Monique Kelly-Kamperdijk

Jemma Kennedy

Misba Khan

Dan Kieran

Alison King

Alice King-Farlow

Hari Kitching

Hilary Knight

Kate Knight

Paula Knight

Helene Kreysa

Titania Krimpas

Tara Lal

Sheila Lamb

Valerie Langfield

Lindi Lawrenson

Fitzroy Lewis

Jonathan Lighthill

Katy Lindemann

Fiona Littleton

Lisa Lloyd

Dood Lloyd-Hughes

Bailey Lock

Mia Loperena

Lyric Hammersmith

James Mackenzie-Blackman

Celina MacManus

Sue Macmillan

Shonaig Macpherson

Lisa Maguire

Linda Malm

Becky Martin

Clare Martin

Eva Martinez Cruz

Sofie Mason

Boris Mavra

Laura McColl

Claire McCormack

Louise McCulloch

Kevin & Kate McGrath

Misty Mcgrath

Joanne McKenna

Ellen McQuaid

Rowan Mead

Emma Middleton

Jane Mitchell

John Mitchinson

Jane Molloy

Carolyn Morris

Tabitha Moses

Alice Moxley

Tomoka Mukai

Rebecca Murray

Carlo Navato

Kirstie Neilson

Rod Newing

Joanna Norland

Louise Norman

Kerry O'Hara

Finola ONeill

Caroline and Sandy Orr

Monica Owsichek

Sophie Paine

Cynthia Painter

Joanne Painter

Rachel Pantin

Anita Pati

Linda Paxton

Caroline Pay

Cathryn Pender

Imogen Perrin

Helen Perrott

Laura Pickard

Jacqui Pickles

Justin Pollard

Caroline Posnansky

Claire Price

Jane Pritchard

Sarah Pullen

Lesley Pyne

Franny Rafferty

Sarah-Jane Rawlings

Susie Ray

Emma Rees

Tina Reid

Jessica Rettie

Julie Ritter

Antonia Rodriguez

Madalyn Roker

Jane Rose

Meriel Rose Whale

Mel Rosenblatt

Geoff Ross

Anthony Ryb

Sarah S

Imogen Sackey

Tracey Sainsbury

Valerie Scarr

Sofia Sciardò

Barbara Scott

Susan Seenan

Natalie Silverman

Anya Sizer

Clive Smith

Rich and Nia Smith

Rima Smith

Sandra Smythe

Katy Snelling

Laura Spoelstra

Sarah Stafford

Anna Stapleton

Victoria Starmer

Jody Stewart

Kitty Stewart

Mandy Stewart

Sharon Straughan

Katy Strudwick

Nina Stutler

Alice Swift Simpkin

Alicja Syska

Andrea Talkenberg

Jaana Tarma

Foy Taylor

Gina Taylor

Alison Telfer

Helen Theofanous

Gillian Thorpe

Dominic Tinley

Abbie Tinsley

Isabelle Titard

Alice Todd

Pamela Mahoney Tsigdinos

Adella Tucker

Becky Turner

Kate Turvey

Vivian van der Kuil

Gabby Vautier

Mauricio Venegas Astorga

Sheree Vickers

Sarah Vilensky

Bridget Ward

Deirdre Ward

Miranda Ward

Suzanna Ward

Wendy Ward

Rachel Watson

Joanne Westwood

Susan Whiddington

Anne Winterbottom

Denise Wood

Emma Wood

Naomi Woolfson

Tracey Woolley

Helen Wright

Stewart Wright